D1326204

Unstable and Brittle Diabetes

Unstable and Brittle Diabetes

Edited by

Geoff Gill

Reader in Medicine & Consultant Physician
University of Liverpool and University Hospital Aintree
Liverpool
UK

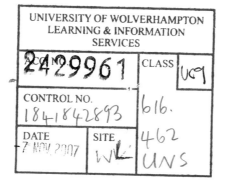

UNIVERSITY OF WOLVERHAMPTON
LEARNING & INFORMATION
SERVICES

ACC NO.	CLASS
2429961	UC9
CONTROL NO.	616.
1841842893	
DATE 7 NOV 2007	SITE WL
	462 UNS

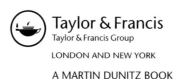

Taylor & Francis
Taylor & Francis Group

LONDON AND NEW YORK

A MARTIN DUNITZ BOOK

© 2004 Taylor & Francis, an imprint of the Taylor & Francis group

First published in the United Kingdom in 2004
by Taylor & Francis, an imprint of the Taylor & Francis Group,
11 New Fetter Lane, London EC4P 4EE

Tel.: +44 (0) 20 7583 9855
Fax.: +44 (0) 20 7842 2298
E-mail: info@dunitz.co.uk
Website: http://www.dunitz.co.uk

All rights reserved. No part of this publication may be reproduced, stored in a
retrieval system, or transmitted, in any form or by any means, electronic,
mechanical, photocopying, recording, or otherwise, without the prior permission of
the publisher or in accordance with the provisions of the Copyright, Designs and
Patents Act 1988 or under the terms of any licence permitting limited copying issued
by the Copyright Licensing Agency, 90 Tottenham Court Road, London W1P 0LP.

Although every effort has been made to ensure that all owners of copyright material
have been acknowledged in this publication, we would be glad to acknowledge in
subsequent reprints or editions any omissions brought to our attention.

A CIP record for this book is available from the British Library.

Library of Congress Cataloging-in-Publication Data

Data available on application

ISBN 1 84184 289 3

Distributed in North and South America by
Taylor & Francis
2000 NW Corporate Blvd
Boca Raton, FL 33431, USA

Within Continental USA
Tel: 800 272 7737; Fax: 800 374 3401
Outside Continental USA
Tel: 561 994 0555; Fax: 561 361 6018
E-mail: orders@crcpress.com

Distributed in the rest of the world by
Thomson Publishing Services
Cheriton House
North Way
Andover, Hampshire SP10 5BE, UK
Tel.: +44 (0)1264 332424
E-mail: salesorder.tandf@thomsonpublishingservices.co.uk

Composition by Scribe Design, Gillingham, Kent
Printed and bound in Great Britain by The Cromwell Press, Trowbridge, Wilts.

Contents

Contents

Contributors

George Alberti
Department of Endocrinology
and Metabolic Medicine,
St Mary's Hospital,
London,
UK

Sue Benbow
Department of Diabetes &
Endocrinology,
University Hospital Aintree,
Liverpool,
UK

Helen Cooper
Department of Primary Care,
University of Liverpool,
Liverpool,
UK

Denise Drumm
Center for Law, Science &
Technology,
Arizona State University,
Tempe, Arizona,
USA,

Jackie Fosbury
Diabetes and Endocrine Day
Centre,
St. Thomas' Hospital,
London ,
UK

Michael Gallagher
Hairmyres Hospital,
East Kilbride,
Scotland,
UK

Geoff Gill
Department of Diabetes &
Endocrinology,
University Hospital Aintree,
Liverpool,
UK

Stephen Greene
Maternal and Child Health
Sciences,
University of Dundee,
Ninewells Hospital,
Dundee,
UK

Elspeth Guthrie
School of Psychiatry &
Behavioural Sciences,
Manchester Royal Infirmary,
Manchester,
UK

Simon Heller
Division of Clinical Sciences,
University of Sheffield,
Sheffield,
UK

Moyyaad Kamali
School of Psychiatry &
Behavioural Sciences,
Manchester Royal Infirmary,
Manchester,
UK

Ray Newton
Postgraduate Medical Office,
Ninewells Hospital and Medical
School,
Dundee,
UK

John Pickup
Metabolic Unit,
Guy's, King's and St Thomas's
School of Medicine,
London,
UK

Jonathan Pinkney
Department of Diabetes &
Endocrinology,
University Hospital Aintree,
Liverpool,
UK

Balasubramanian Ravikumar
Diabetes Research Centre,
The Medical School,
University of Newcastle,
Newcastle-upon-Tyne,
UK

David Schade
Division of Endocrinology &
Metabolism,
University of New Mexico,
Albuquerque,
New Mexico,
USA

Robert Tattersall
Curzon House,
Curzon Street,
Gotham,
Nottingham,
UK

Roy Taylor
Department of Medicine,
Royal Victoria Infirmary,
Newcastle upon Tyne,
UK

John Wilding
Department of Diabetes &
Endocrinology,
University Hospital Aintree,
Liverpool,
UK

Gareth Williams
Dean's Office,
Faculy of Medicine & Dentistry,
University of Bristol,
Bristol,
UK

Series preface

Advances in Diabetes is a new series of monographs, each concerned with a hot or rapidly-evolving topic in diabetes. Our understanding of the processes involved in diabetes advances at the same time as new treatments emerge. There is a space for an up-to-date series of concise texts which outline these advances and this series is aimed at specialist medical and nursing practitioners in diabetes, together with their trainees. I hope that you find this series useful and stimulating as it brings together the latest information on each topic under review.

H Jonathan Bodansky
The General Infirmary at Leeds, Leeds, UK

Preface

Both sub-groups of diabetes mellitus – types 1 and 2 – are, for different reasons, difficult or impossible to adequately control. Diabetes health professionals regularly have to compromise ideal glycaemic aims against what can reasonably be achieved with the imperfect tools of our trade, and the ever-present battle for patient-compliance. There are, however, extremes of control difficulty. In type 1 diabetes, such patients are frequently termed "brittle". They defy any semblance of metabolic control and are recurrently hospitalized with hyperglycaemic or hypoglycaemic crises. The very term "brittle" is shrouded in mystery as to its origin and in controversy as to its usefulness.

This is the first book for nearly 20 years to deal with the problem of severely unstable diabetes. As well as brittle type 1 syndromes, the scope of instability has been extended to the notoriously problematic issue of obese and highly insulin-resistant type 2 diabetes, as well as instability in special groups such as the very young and the elderly. A multi-disciplinary and highly experienced group of writers have contributed, and there is even a final chapter by a patient. Issues of psychology, psychiatry and education are included, as well as more "medical" forms of management, such as insulin pump therapy and pancreas transplantation. The aim is to provide a balanced view of this most difficult area of diabetes care.

Geoff Gill
Liverpool, UK

chapter 1

Unstable and brittle diabetes: past and present

Robert Tattersall

The success or failure of diabetic control is largely dependent upon the active participation of the patient in treatment, and his or her use of discerning judgement in unusual situations not specifically covered by physician instruction. Obviously, this places far more responsibility for the maintenance of disease control on the patient than is true of most other diseases.[1]

The inability or wilful refusal of the sick to follow their doctor's recommendations is not new. In the second edition of his famous book in 1798, John Rollo recorded the case of a 57-year-old general who was treated successfully by dietary restriction but returned to apple puddings and wine and died within 3 months. He was an example of what Frederick Allen, of undernutrition treatment fame, described as 'the habitually unfaithful type of patient.'[2] Shrewdly, Allen pointed out that 'fidelity' could not be predicted from any criteria of intelligence or social position – a lesson which would frequently be forgotten by those dealing with difficult to control diabetes over the next 80 years.[3] Then, as now, doctors had to work with the material they were given and Allen claimed that the 96 patients he treated with undernutrition between 1914 and 1917, 'ranged from the ignorant shiftless poor to the pampered willful rich'.[4]

1

The first 15 years after the introduction of insulin

When insulin was first used in 1922–3, anyone with a knowledge of human nature would have predicted that a treatment which was, at least in theory, under the patient's control, would lead to trouble in some cases. Surprisingly, in the euphoria following its introduction, problems of compliance do not seem to have been anticipated, possibly because of the authoritarian zeitgeist of the time, but more likely because it was thought that those who had been saved from certain death would repay the discoverers of insulin by making the most of their reprieve.

Another important point is that physicians of the time had no training in the management of chronic disease. Brought up on physical signs and acute illnesses, they were basically detectives whose work was finished when the crime was solved. Most did not see continuing care and support as part of their remit. It soon became clear that trying to keep the urine sugar free was an arduous task and the few 24-hour blood sugar profiles which were done before World War II showed wide fluctuations from hyper- to hypoglycaemia and back again.[5] Most diabetes specialists attributed lability of blood sugar levels to the imperfect pharmacodynamics of insulin, a problem which had become worse with increasing purification in the late 1920s when insulin became 'almost explosive in its action.'[6] The term 'brittle diabetes' was apparently introduced in the 1930s by the Chicago physician Rollin T Woodyatt (1878–1953), although no-one has been able to find the citation. The earliest reference I have found is in Woodyatt's colleague Russell Wilder's 1940 textbook where he wrote:

> In addition, there is a group of patients with unusually
> unstable blood sugar levels with whom everyone with
> experience of diabetes has run into difficulties. Woodyatt has
> labeled them 'brittle cases'. The patient passes rapidly from
> the condition of hyperglycemia, even with acidosis, to

hypoglycemia and back again. Such patients require most careful management and with them *severe reactions* can be avoided only by accepting some degree of under-treatment and carefully avoiding aglycosuric urine.[7] [my italics]

From Wilder's reference to severe reactions, it sounds as though the crux of brittleness was frequent hypoglycaemia. Nevertheless, some patients did become seriously ill from ketoacidosis at regular intervals; a child in Boston had 19 episodes between 1925 and her death in coma at age 16 in 1931. Apart from commenting that 'it is rather extraordinary for a patient to have been in diabetic coma and to have recovered from it on 19 occasions' and that she did not follow her diet, the paper gives no explanation or hypothesis for why this should have happened.[8] Perhaps there was no need because most physicians would have dismissed it as the result of 'ignorance and folly'.[9] In 1937, Elliott Joslin, arguably the most famous diabetes specialist of the twentieth century, wrote:

> The treatment of diabetes is so successful today that when unsatisfactory results are obtained, the whole situation should be investigated anew to determine the cause ... one must remember that diabetes is a good disease which often has bad companions, whose *medical* identity must be sought and fought.[10] [my italics]

These 'bad companions' were exclusively medical and consisted of conditions such as thyrotoxicosis, tuberculosis or occult infections. Joslin never mentions emotional problems or non-compliance, probably because, as a New England Puritan, such 'weaknesses' were not part of his vocabulary. A possible explanation of brittleness was that it was due to overactivity of other endocrine glands, particularly the pituitary and adrenal. On the basis of this hypothesis, some patients were subjected to bilateral splanchnic nerve section[11] or pituitary radiotherapy.[12]

Psychoanalysts enter the field

As [predominantly Jewish] psychoanalysts were driven out of their Germanic homelands from the early 1930s, they emigrated to the USA, where they had a major influence on psychiatry and brought with them the new specialty of psychosomatic medicine, a reaction to what its founders saw as the takeover of medicine by technology and the laboratory. Psychoanalysts were highly critical of physicians who looked after diabetic patients. In 1935, William Menninger wrote that:

> The lack of description of psychopathology in diabetics by internists may, in part, be explained by their interest in treating the disease and not the person. Consequently, unless the patient emphasises his mental difficulties, no notice or investigation of the field is usually made.[13]

When another psychoanalyst, George Daniels, searched *Index Medicus* between 1934 and 1939, he found 3333 articles on diabetes of which only 23 had titles calling attention to emotional problems; most of these were about whether nervous shocks could cause the disease. According to him:

> Except in the articles definitely written from the psychological or psychiatric viewpoint, even the subject of fluctuations in the disease due to emotional change – of which almost every physician is aware – is not re-emphasised nor included with any regularity among the complications of the disease. One gathers that this is partly because it is not fully appreciated and partly because it is thought of as being unscientific.[14]

Emotional stress as a cause of lability: 1939–50

Between 1939 and 1950 a trickle of papers documented the high prevalence of psychological problems among diabetic patients,

4

especially children. At the American Psychiatric Association meeting in 1939, Shirley and Greer concluded that diabetes in childhood was often complicated by 'unsound economic conditions, unwholesome home environments, faulty parental attitudes, and poor cooperation and handicapping reactions on the part of the child.'[15] In 1944 Loughlin and Mosenthal found that a third of children with recurrent ketoacidosis came from broken homes and many freely admitted that they preferred hospital to home.[16] In 1946, Fischer and Dolger reported 43 diabetic children from poor or lower middle class homes followed for 10–20 years and emphasized the frequency of psychological problems.[17]

One of the most striking papers in this period is that of Harold Rosen and Theodore Lidz – the latter the first psychoanalyst on the staff of Johns Hopkins – who interviewed 12 patients who each had an average of 5.5 admissions with ketoacidosis.[18] The physician believed that they had 'metabolic eccentricities which made them react severely to slight changes in diet, insulin intake, exercise, or general health', but Rosen and Lidz found that all had deliberately disrupted their diabetes to escape from difficulties either by flight into hospital or by trying to end their own lives. This did not simplify treatment, but knowing that they did not just 'slip into acidosis', had led, according to the authors, to less concern about the minutiae of their regulation. They comment that, 'despite the gross instability of personality organisation apparent in all the patients, few suffered from psychiatric syndromes that could be readily classified.'

In 1946, Arthur Mirsky, a biochemist who later trained as a psychoanalyst,[19] showed that hyperglycaemia could be induced by stress interviews.[20] Another psychoanalyst, Lawrence Hinkle, working at Edward Tolstoi's clinic in New York, continued this line of investigation with an in-depth study of three people with labile diabetes. Their life histories were obtained in detailed interviews totalling 20 or 30 hours over 1 or 2 years.[21] These were unashamedly psychoanalytical: for example, dreams were discussed and attention paid to 'slips of the tongue, things said, and things left unsaid'. The three subjects, aged 19, 21 and 38, all had severely labile diabetes and chaotic and complicated private lives. For each subject, Hinkle et al charted the clinical course, as measured by glycosuria and ketonuria, alongside significant life events. They acknowledged that the connection between stress and ketonuria need not be direct, writing that:

> Patients usually react to stressful life situations with alterations of their total behaviour. In addition to the direct metabolic changes which take place it is quite customary for them to alter their eating habits, neglect to sterilize their equipment, and take their insulin irregularly, partially, or not at all, during stressful episodes. All of these factors work together to cause ketosis and coma.

Recurrent ketoacidosis

Cases of repeated or tautologous ketoacidosis occurred in all countries where there was insulin-dependent diabetes. At the second conference of the International Diabetes Federation, held in Cambridge, England in 1955, the Pecks (father and son) reported a woman with almost 50 admissions in 8 years, and physicians from Australia, Holland, Northern Ireland and England had all seen cases where the number of admissions was well into double figures.[22] The Pecks' patient was 'cured' by taking her away from her alcoholic criminal mother and giving her a sheltered job in the hospital kitchen. However, by the mid 1950s, a situation had arisen, especially in the USA, where one group of doctors believed that unknown endogenous factors caused unpredictable swings in blood glucose between hypoglycaemia and ketoacidosis while another group attributed the same phenomena to emotional upsets and deliberate sabotage of treatment. Even the latter group were divided into those who believed that the emotions acted through unconscious mechanisms and those who thought the patients deliberately punished themselves.

Two panel discussions published in *Diabetes* illustrate the schism. At the annual meeting of the American Diabetes Association in 1956, the moderator Alexander Marble of the Joslin Clinic rejected the adjective 'brittle' in favour of 'labile' or 'insulin sensitive', and put the crucial question: 'Are we talking about diabetes that is unstable, or about a diabetic person who is unstable?'[23] Garfield Duncan of Philadelphia thought the problem was basically emotional and his suggested solution was that the internist should take a full psychiatric history; in particular, he made the simple suggestion that 'the home situation should be gone into in detail'. Alexander Marble summed up with his view that it was all a matter of inappropriate treatment, and that even patients with the most unstable form of diabetes could be regulated with careful attention to diet and exercise. Three years later, in 1959, *Diabetes* published a debate from a New York symposium on 'The role of environment and personality in the management of the difficult patient with diabetes mellitus.' The chairman, psychiatrist Lawrence Hinkle, suggested provocatively that physicians could not cope with 'difficult diabetics' because they did not take proper histories and did not maintain a non-punitive attitude. According to him, they were:

> Unable or unwilling to view disturbances of mood, thought,
> and behaviour with a detached and clinical eye. All too often,
> they regard these manifestations of the patient's illness –
> which in truth may be boundlessly annoying – as personal
> affronts, and as soon as their own emotions become involved
> they lose their effectiveness as physicians.[24]

Finding out about a patient's life situation and background was, according to Hinkle, easy: 'One simply asks the patient. After all he came to a physician and he expects to be asked questions.' How the questions were phrased was important. Somewhat patronisingly, Hinkle pointed out that, 'Naturally, if one asks him, does he love his mother? or, does he get along with his wife? The answer will be "yes".' In another paper Hinkle suggested that physicians needed 'infinite patience, adult wisdom, sympathetic understanding, and a friendly, reasonable, but firm failure to approve of irrational rebellion.'[25] He ended by saying that:

Treatment directed at the individual, at his environment, and at his attitudes and feelings toward it may diminish or even abolish such fluctuations [of blood sugar]. Such treatment may be difficult and time consuming, but simple manipulation of diet and insulin can never be more than palliative in such cases, and is often quite futile.

Where did this leave the average physician in 1960? Were there, as suggested in the published discussions, two separate groups of patients: one with lability which could be cured by adjusting the insulin, diet and exercise, and another where the lability was of emotional origin? Did the 'insulinologists' have patients they had never reported in whom the instability was clearly of emotional origin? Or was it that when psychoanalysts were let loose on diabetic patients, they were bound to uncover psychic traumas which were irrelevant to the problem of lability? The debate had become so polarized that nobody knew. Also, there was no forum to continue the debate because psychosomatic medicine itself was in crisis.[26] What had originally started as a movement to integrate somatic therapy and psychotherapy had been abandoned, even by those physicians and surgeons who had originally been interested. Worse still, the psychoanalysts had become discouraged. At the end of his presidential address to the American Psychosomatic Society in 1960, Eric Wittkower asked rhetorically, 'Is it really true that we have struggled in vain for so many years and that the contributions made by psychoanalysts amount to nil?' Many diabetes specialists would doubtless have answered, 'Yes'.

Back to biochemistry: 1960–75

By the mid 1960s radioimmunoassay had made it possible to measure insulin and other hormones. Continuous blood glucose analysis gave a more comprehensive picture of between- and within-day fluctuations from which various mathematical measures of instability could be derived, such as the 'M value' of Jørgen Schlichtkrull of Copenhagen. Between 1960 and 1974 the task of quantitating brittleness was most enthusiastically undertaken by the Canadian physician George Molnar and his associates at the Mayo Clinic. Starting from an intensive study of one patient, they suggested that the characteristics of hyperlabile diabetes could be described 'on the basis of clinical experience and by the study in depth of some prototypical patients'.[27] How one recognized prototypical patients was not made clear, but the defining factor was unexpected and unpredictable hypoglycaemic reactions. Patient or physician error had to be excluded by a 'rigorous and usually prolonged trial of therapy'. The lack of any details about Molnar's patients apart from age, duration of diabetes and insulin regimens is in sharp contrast to Hinkle's elaborate tables showing how metabolic decompensation coincided with adverse life events and moods.

A 30-year-old farmer was the only subject in two long papers from the Mayo Clinic. For 142 days he was studied continuously in a metabolic ward, where he 'subsisted on a weighed, balance study type of diet and ate, slept, and exercised by the clock. Specimens of urine were tested and samples of excreta were collected, similarly by the clock'.[28] The main conclusion was that four times daily insulin produced good control, which deteriorated when he returned to one injection. With him and other patients, Molnar and colleagues tried a variety of manoeuvres and therapies, including exercise, phenformin and nicotinic acid. Further attempts at mathematical expression of brittleness resulted in 'MAGE' or the **M**ean **A**mplitude of **G**lycaemic **E**xcursions. In patients with 'hyperlabile' diabetes, MAGE had an irreducible minimum, in that intensification of insulin therapy reduced the nadirs as well as glycaemic peaks and so increased the frequency of hypoglycaemia. All Molnar's patients were said to have been evaluated by 'a battery of psychological tests and psychiatric interviews', and he concluded that unstable diabetes was due to factors other than lack of patient cooperation or inadequate treatment. Among the putative causes were excessive growth hormone and abnormal glucagon secretion, although what correlated best with the degree of lability was the severity of insulin deficiency.

Other causes which were strongly considered during this period were insulin antibodies and the Somogyi effect.

Insulin antibodies

Most patients up to the 1970s had moderate titres of insulin antibodies that were considered important because they made insulin less effective, and, in extreme cases, led to insulin resistance. In many patients antibodies were 'good' in the sense that they had a 'smoothing' effect in prolonging the effects of exogenous insulin.[29] In effect, they made soluble insulin last as long as isophane, which is why many patients could be satisfactorily treated with twice-daily soluble insulin. In 1972, Dixon et al from Birmingham, England compared 6 patients with labile diabetes and 13 who were stable. Patients in the labile group had very small amounts of antibody or antibodies that were avid binders of insulin, whereas the stable group had moderate amounts of insulin-binding antibodies of low affinity.[30] This work began at the time when new highly purified insulins were being introduced and probably fizzled out because it was not in the interest of the insulin manufacturers to fund it. Nevertheless, it remains true that instability, particularly hypoglycaemic brittleness, can often be cured by eschewing multiple injections of fast-acting insulin in favour of two or three injections of a long-acting one, preferably of animal origin.

The Somogyi effect

The idea behind the Somogyi effect was that hypoglycaemia (often asymptomatic and at night) stimulated the release of counter-regulatory hormones, which caused rebound hyperglycaemia.[31] It was taken up in a big way, especially by paediatricians in the USA, as *the* explanation for fasting hyperglycaemia. The standard explanation for a high blood sugar first thing in the morning was that the child 'must have

Somogyied during the night'. Eventually it was shown that Somogyi's concept of an exaggerated counter-regulatory response was wrong and that fasting hyperglycaemia was caused by a fall in free insulin concentration overnight.[32] Again, the solution is a longer-acting basal insulin with as little peak as possible.

History repeats itself

Woodyatt's definition was thought to embrace about 10% of all type 1 diabetic patients, which I felt was unhelpful, since many of those thereby labelled 'brittle' led reasonably normal lives. Indeed, some were only unmasked by 24-hour glucose profiles. I felt that a more restrictive definition would be more useful to clinicians and in 1977 I tried to reconcile the biochemical and psychological camps by defining the brittle diabetic as one 'whose life is constantly disrupted by episodes of hypo- or hyperglycaemia whatever their cause.'[33] It was clear that there were 'obviously organic' causes such as Addison's disease and coeliac disease, but these generally caused recurrent hypoglycaemia. By contrast, a convincing organic cause of recurrent episodes of ketoacidosis was hardly ever found. My experience recalled John Malin's comment that 'Conversation with some of these reformed characters is instructive as they reveal the extent of their deviations from the prescribed treatment'.[34] I wrote that:

> No series has so far been the subject of a systematic
> psychiatric survey and it is impossible to know how often
> emotional disturbance in a less dramatic form [than that of the
> Pecks' patient with tautologous ketoacidosis] is the
> precipitating factor. It must be emphasized that even where
> ketoacidosis has been self induced, patients may offer
> superficially plausible explanations for the loss of diabetic
> control and it may be very time consuming to uncover the
> emotional cause.

Technology to the rescue

At the end of the 1970s, the pattern of normal insulin secretion was known and could be mimicked with infusions and pumps. If the problem was one of insulin delivery, it seemed that it should be possible to stabilize even the most difficult patients. Two English groups – at Guy's Hospital, London, and the Freeman Hospital, Newcastle – took up the challenge and collected relatively homogeneous cohorts of young women with recurrent ketoacidosis. Thirteen patients 'disabled by unpredictable metabolic swings' were studied at Guy's Hospital, London in 1980–3. All were tertiary referrals and all were females between the ages of 13 and 35 who were unresponsive to continuous subcutaneous insulin infusion (CSII). Eight patients were treated with long-term continuous intravenous insulin infusion, but the results were unsatisfactory in seven patients and it was discontinued because of serious complications. At follow-up of these women in 1987 the number of hospital admissions, as well as total insulin doses, had fallen substantially but all but one were still metabolically unstable. What had also become apparent was that:

> Episodes of non-compliance were detected or suspected in
> eight ... some episodes were *relatively minor* (e.g.
> immobilising infusion pumps by inverting or removing the
> batteries, eating binges, feigning hypoglycaemia, faking insulin
> injections), while more serious interference with treatment
> included cutting intravenous infusion lines, diluting
> intravenously infused insulin with tap water, and apparent self-
> exsanguination through a central venous catheter. [my italics]

A similar group of young women was studied in Newcastle where it was thought that 'the stereotyped clinical characteristics suggested a new diabetic syndrome possibly with a biochemical basis'. A number of possibilities, including defective insulin absorption, degradation of insulin at the injection site, inappropriate secretion of glucagon, growth hormone, and catecholamines, accelerated ketogenesis, etc., were investigated, but eventually it became clear that many patients were interfering with therapy. It was then suggested that self-induced instability might lead to a vicious cycle in which the patient became locked into an acquired metabolic problem. Of the 26 patients who could be traced for follow-up between 1991 and 1993, 5 had died, but of the 21 survivors only 2 were still considered brittle.

At the same time as the Newcastle and Guy's studies, David Schade and colleagues in New Mexico investigated 30 patients (23 female) from all over the USA, who, in spite of intensified insulin therapy, were unable to stay out of hospital long enough to lead anything approaching a normal life. Using an algorithmic approach Schade found that 8 patients had factitious disease, 8 were malingering, 7 had what he called 'communication disorders' and only 6 had recognized organic causes for their extreme brittleness. Factitious disease was defined as interference with treatment and it is of interest that in 4 patients the correct diagnosis was made not by the doctors, but by nurses on the clinical research unit.

Schade et al pointed out, as many had done before, that one reason for missing factitious disease was that the relationship of the physician (and nurses) to the patient was so close that the possibility was never considered. Even when it had been proved, the referring physicians of 3 of Schade's patients refused to accept it. In a detailed description of 5 cases, Schade et al note that, while an intelligent patient may avoid being 'caught' during a short observation period (especially in an ordinary hospital ward), continuing surveillance will eventually provide the diagnosis. This, of course, assumes that the physician remembers Sherlock Holmes' comment to the hapless Dr Watson, 'How often have I said to you that when you have eliminated the possible, what remains, *however improbable*, must be the truth.'[35]

Overlooked groups

Research based on tertiary referral series leads to stereotyping because the referring physicians give the researchers what they think they want (or what they, the referrers, want to get rid of). Thus, it became accepted that brittle diabetes was the preserve of young women. However, in a 12-year follow-up of unselected patients with brittle diabetes in Nottingham, I found that nearly half the patients were men.[36] When thinking about this, my mind went back to a patient who held the record for the number of admissions with ketoacidosis at King's College Hospital, London, when I worked there in the early 1970s. Everybody knew that he induced ketoacidosis to get away from his wicked stepfather or, if he had been thrown out of home, to get a bed and care for a few days. He was never called a brittle diabetic and nobody would have dreamed of referring him to Guy's or Newcastle for further investigation. On the other hand, there were several young women in the same clinic whose instability was thoroughly mysterious.

The idea that instability was confined to the young was challenged by a paper published in 1989 which reported 6 cases of severely unstable diabetes in the elderly.[37] In a questionnaire survey in 1996, Gill and colleagues found that most physicians knew of at least one similar elderly patient.[38] In their series of 55, the mean age was 74 and the mean duration of diabetes 24 years, 70% were female; 22 (44%) had mixed brittleness, 16 (29%) recurrent diabetic ketoacidosis (DKA) and 15 (27%) recurrent hypoglycaemia.

A new cause of brittle diabetes which emerged in the 1980s was eating disorders.[39] The main reason for the delayed recognition of what may always have been a relatively common cause of poor diabetic control or brittleness is that most remain in the diabetic clinic where they are conspicuous for their high blood glucose levels, but nobody thinks to ask why with such awful control they do not lose weight. It is now clear that omission of doses of insulin, for whatever reason, is common among young people with type 1 diabetes.[40]

Personal memories

In his book entitled *Who Has Seen a Blood Sugar?*, Frank Davidoff, when considering how to deal with uninteresting or demanding patients, suggests that the way to make diabetes interesting is to learn 'what makes these individual patients "tick," biologicially and psychologically; figuring out how best to interact with each of them; deciding how best to negotiate, to develop therapeutic alliances, to use language effectively – all provide endless sources of interest.' My first and last patients with brittle diabetes illustrate this well.

Patient 1 (solved in 1971)

This woman with hypoglycaemic brittleness was the diabetic member of a pair of discordant identical twins. She had never been in hospital in 30 years of diabetes but constantly complained of inability to achieve stable control together with frequent hypoglycaemia. When she came to the clinic, she baffled the doctors with her urine testing charts, which, because they were in the colours of Clinitest, resembled Rubik's cube. When I visited her at home as part of our research, I was surprised to be told to take off my shoes as I crossed the threshold. To cut a long story short, it transpired that she was obsessional not only about tidiness and cleanliness but also about her diabetes. If her morning urine test showed sugar, she got into a panic, did not have breakfast but tested an hour later. If the second test showed sugar, she went for a run 'to burn it off'. This often led to hypoglycaemia, which forced her to eat, led to sugar in the pre-lunch urine test, and caused the whole cycle to repeat itself. It appeared that 20 years earlier, a doctor who was frustrated at her lack of control had told her never to change the insulin dose!

Patient 2 (solved in 1996)

This girl developed diabetes at age 8 and was stable until she started menstruating at age 12, when recurrent ketoacidosis began with admissions every other month. The diabetes nurse specialist and I held several meetings with the family – father, mother, the patient and her younger sister – but could never get any admission of anything wrong. Because the girl was hardly ever at school, I arranged for her to board at a special school for 'delicate' children run by the County Council. This was a great success; her insulin dose halved, urine tests for ketones became negative and she was never ill – except when she came home for weekends and holidays. We dreaded the day when she would reach school leaving age – rightly, because in the first year she had 18 admissions with ketoacidosis. It seemed obvious that the problem must be at home and, educated by the Cleveland Inquiry, we suspected sexual abuse. Eventually the girl asked to see the diabetes specialist nurse and revealed that her father had been sexually abusing her since the age of 12 and that she had not felt able to tell anyone.

Is the concept of brittle diabetes useful?

In 1963, the New York diabetologist Harold Rifkin wrote that 'we have been cautioned in the past against the use of the term "brittle diabetic" since it has been claimed that it is more frequently the attending physician who is "brittle" rather than his patient'.[41] Certainly it is not useful for the admitting doctor to write 'well-known brittle diabetic', the implication being that this is a diagnosis. It is equally unhelpful for patients to announce triumphantly on their first visit to a new clinic that 'Dr X told me years ago that I am a brittle diabetic', the implication being that they should be left alone and allowed to seek refuge in hospital if things overwhelm them in the outside world.

I do think using the adjective 'brittle' to characterize two ends of a very wide spectrum is useful, provided people realize that it is no more a diagnosis than 'jaundice' or 'anaemia'. It is also necessary to stress that life disruption does not have to include hospital admissions; severe hypoglycaemic brittleness is often concealed at home where the spouse resignedly accepts it as 'one of those things'.

Once a patient has been labelled 'brittle', a diagnosis is vital for future management. How such a diagnosis can be (hopefully) made will be covered by other contributors in this book, but it should be emphasized that recurrent hypoglycaemia and recurrent DKA are different conditions with different prognoses. The former condition is more likely to be organic, and the latter behavioural.

References

1. Palmer RW. The diabetic personality. J Indiana Med Assoc 1958; 51: 1399.
2. Allen FM, Sherrill JW. Clinical observations with insulin. J Metab Res 1922; 2: 803–95.
3. Steel JM. Such a nice girl. Lancet 1994; 344: 365–6.
4. Allen FM, Stillman E, Fitz R. Total dietary regulation in the treatment of diabetes. The Rockefeller Institute for Medical Research, Monograph No. 11, New York, 1919.
5. Maddock SJ, Trimble HC. Prolonged insulin hypoglycemia without symptoms. J Am Med Assoc 1928; 91: 616–21. See also: Sprague PH, Newson DA. A study of the twenty four hour blood sugar curve in diabetic patients. Canad Med Assoc J 1934; 609–11.
6. Campbell WR, Fletcher AA, Kerr RB. Protamine insulin in the treatment of diabetes mellitus. Trans Ass Am Phys 1936; 51: 161–73.
7. Wilder RM. Clinical diabetes and hyperinsulinism. WB Saunders, Philadelphia, 1940, pp 100–1.
8. Ralli EP, Waterhouse AM. Diabetic coma occurring 19 times in the life of a patient with diabetes mellitus. J Lab Clin Med 1933; 18: 1119–27.
9. Baker TW. A clinical survey of one hundred and eight consecutive cases of diabetic coma. Arch Int Med 1936; 58: 373–406.
10. Joslin EP. The treatment of diabetes mellitus, 6th edn. Henry Kimpton, London, 1937, p 264.
11. De Takats G. Splanchnic nerve section in juvenile diabetes. Ann Int Med 1934; 7: 1201–17.
12. Pollack H. In discussion of McCullagh EP. Diabetogenic action of the pituitary: clinical observations. Diabetes 1956; 5: 33–4.
13. Menninger WC. The inter-relationship of mental disorders and diabetes mellitus. J Ment Sci 1935; 81: 332–57.
14. Daniels GE. Present trends in the evaluation of psychic factors in diabetes mellitus. Psychosom Med 1939; 1: 527–52.
15. Shirley HF, Greer IM. Environmental and personality problems in the treatment of diabetic children. J Pediat 1943; 16: 775–81.
16. Loughlin WC, Mosenthal HO. Study of the personalities of children with diabetes. Am J Dis Child 1944; 68: 13–15.
17. Fischer AE, Dolger H. Behavior and psychologic problems of young diabetic patients. Arch Int Med 1946; 78: 711–31.
18. Rosen H, Lidz T. Emotional factors in the precipitation of recurrent diabetic acidosis. Psychosom Med 1949; 11: 211–15.
19. In Memoriam. I Arthur Mirsky, MD, 1907–74. Psychosom Med 1975; 37: 1–3. See also: Danowski TS, Hofmann KI. Arthur Mirsky, 1907–1974. Diabetes 1975; 24: 776–8.
20. Mirsky IA. Emotional hyperglycaemia. Proc Central Soc Clin Res 1946; 19: 75.
21. Hinkle LE, Evans FM, Wolf S. Studies in diabetes mellitus. III. Life history of three persons with labile diabetes and relation of significant experiences in their lives to the onset and course of the disease. Psychosom Med 1950; 13: 160–83.

22. Peck FB Sr, Peck FB Jr. Tautologous diabetic coma – a behavior syndrome. Diabetes 1956; 5: 45–8.
23. Panel discussion: Unstable diabetes. Diabetes 1956; 5: 475–83.
24. Hinkle LE, Knowles HC, Fischer A, Stunkard AJ. Role of environment and personality in management of the difficult patient with diabetes mellitus. Diabetes 1959; 8: 371–82.
25. Hinkle LE. The doctor–patient relationship in the management of diabetic patients and their emotional problems. New York State J Med 1953; 53: 1943–5.
26. Wittkower ED. Twenty years of North American Psychosomatic Medicine. Psychosom Med 1960; 22: 308–16.
27. Molnar GD, Gastineau CF, Rosevear JW, Moxness KE. Quantitative aspects of labile diabetes. Diabetes 1965; 14; 279–88.
28. Molnar GD, McGuckin WF, Striebel JL, Gastineau CF. Effects of therapeutic measures in a hyperlabile diabetic. Proc Staff Meet Mayo Clinic 1961; 36: 45–61. See also: Molnar GD, Gastineau CF, Rosevear JW et al. Metabolic effects of exercise and multiple-dose insulin regimens in hyperlabile diabetes mellitus. Metabolism 1963; 12: 157–63.
29. Palumbo PJ, Taylor WF, Molnar GD, Tauxe WN. Disappearance of bovine insulin from plasma in normal and diabetic subjects. Metabolism 1972; 21: 787–98.
30. Dixon K, Exon PD, Hughes HR. Insulin antibodies in the aetiology of labile diabetes. Lancet 1972; 1: 343–7.
31. Much of the information in this section is taken from Gale EAM. The Somogyi effect. In: Nattrass M, ed., Recent advances in diabetes, 2nd edn. Churchill Livingstone, Edinburgh, 1986.
32. Gale EAM, Tattersall RB. Unrecognised nocturnal hypoglycaemia in insulin-treated diabetics. Lancet 1979; 1: 1049–52. See also: Gale EAM, Kurtz AB, Tattersall RB. In search of the Somogyi effect. Lancet 1980; 2: 279–82.
33. Tattersall R. Brittle diabetes. Clin Endocrinol Metab 1977; 6: 403–19.
34. Malins JM. Clinical diabetes mellitus. Eyre and Spottiswoode, London, 1968, pp 107–8.
35. Conan Doyle AC. The sign of four. Spencer Blackett, London, 1890.
36. Tattersall RB, Gregory R, Heller SR et al. The natural history of brittle diabetes: a 12 year follow up. Br Med J 1991; 302: 1240–3.
37. Griffith DNW, Yudkin J. Brittle diabetes in the elderly. Diabet Med 1989; 6: 440–3.
38. Gill GV, Lucas S, Kent LA. Prevalence and characteristics of brittle diabetes in Britain. Q J Med 1996; 89: 839–43.
39. Steel JM, Young RJ, Lloyd GG, MacIntyre CCA. Abnormal eating attitudes in young insulin-dependent diabetics. Br J Psychiatry 1989; 515–21.
40. Morris AD, Boyle DIR, McMahon AD et al. Adherence to insulin treatment, glycaemic control and ketoacidosis in insulin-dependent diabetes mellitus. Lancet 1997; 350: 1505–10.
41. Rifkin H. Clinical impact of insulin. Diabetes 1963; 12: 31–7.

chapter 2

An overview of brittle diabetes

Geoff Gill and Gareth Williams

This chapter will attempt to bring together the many diverse strands of research into 'brittleness' in type 1 diabetes. Our aim is to give a reasonably objective overview of the current status of the condition in terms of definition, prevalence and characteristics, aetiology and outcome. We will also explore the status of brittleness as an extreme end of a spectrum which merges into the vast number of imperfectly controlled and 'unstable' patients with type 1 diabetes.

Defining brittle diabetes

One of the reasons why brittle diabetes remains a contentious area of diabetology is the difficulty and disagreement over its definition. This has not been helped by the persistent mis-referencing of the original definition, supposedly originating from the American physician Rollin Woodyatt. This was said to be:

> insulin-dependent diabetes whose control is so fragile that
> they are subject to frequent and precipitous fluctuations
> between hyperglycaemia and insulin reactions, and in whom
> other causes of instability have been excluded.

This apparently precise definition was widely quoted, and referenced to *Cecil's Textbook of Medicine* in various years during the 1930s (when Woodyatt did in fact write the diabetes section of the book).[1] In 1988, Schade drew attention to difficulties in locating this quote,[2] and 3 years later we also recorded our own failures of location in a more extensive search.[3] Robert Tattersall's detailed historical researches[4] found that the earliest use of the Woodyatt reference was in 1950,[5] and from then on future generations of 'brittle diabetologists' continually misquoted this reference as a 'self-replicating bibliographic virus'![3] Tattersall also found that the earliest use of the term 'brittle' was in Wilder's textbook *Clinical Diabetes and Hyperinsulinism* of 1940.[6] Here, Wilder again emphasizes the concept of glycaemic fluctuations ('acidosis to hypoglycaemia and back again'), and stated that 'Woodyatt has labelled them brittle cases'. Tattersall believes that the name and concept of brittle diabetes was introduced by Woodyatt sometime in the 1930s as an oral rather than written description.

Whatever its origins, the idea that brittleness was associated with glycaemic swings persisted, and was again emphasized by Molnar in 1964.[7] However, the definition became increasingly unsatisfactory, and indeed, retrospectively, may have been related to the popularity of single-dose long-acting insulins, for example PZI (or protamine-zinc insulin), which notoriously caused glycaemic peaks and troughs. The original concept also ignored a small group of patients with arguably the most difficult form of instability – those with recurrent diabetic ketoacidosis (DKA). This syndrome had been recognized since its description by Rosen and Lidz in 1949.[8] Because of these problems, in 1977 Tattersall suggested a broader definition which accepted any type of glycaemic instability. He proposed that brittle diabetes be redefined as 'the patient whose life is constantly being disrupted by episodes of hypo- or hyperglycaemia whatever their cause'.[9] Though open to some criticism, and subjected to later adaptations, this concept of brittle type 1 diabetes has largely persisted to the present.

However, despite its general acceptance, the definition is subjective, and as researchers attempted to investigate brittle diabetes scientifically in the 1980s and 1990s, more objective definitions were

Table 2.1 Some subjective and objective definitions of severe glycaemic instability or 'brittleness' in type 1 diabetes

Definition	Reference
Subjective:	
'Life disruption due to hypo- or hyperglycaemia of any cause'	Tattersall[9]
'Severe glycaemic instability unresponsive to intensified subcutaneous insulin therapy'	Pickup et al[13]
'Severe glycaemic instability with life disruption and repeated and/or prolonged hospitalisations'	Gill et al[11]
Objective:	
'Either incapacitated, or life disrupted more than 3 times per week by repeated hypo- or hyperglycaemia'	Schade[2]
'At least 3 hospitalisations with either hypo- or hyperglycaemia in a two year period'	Tattersall et al[10]

introduced, mostly attempting to quantify episodes of life disruption or metabolic decompensation. Two of these are shown in Table 2.1, and it can be seen that even Tattersall's group adopted a numerical definition for one of their investigations.[10] Though such objective definitions clearly have advantages, they still depend on events which may not have agreed definitions (e.g. 'incapacitation' or 'life disruption').[2] Even when events are clearly definable (e.g. hospitalization[10]) the number of such events required for the diagnosis of brittleness may be debatable. For this reason, other workers have retained subjective definitions, sometimes adapting the original Tattersall concept. Gill and colleagues added the requirement of 'recurrent and/or repeated hospitalizations' to life disruption.[11] The wording is important, as some patients with recurrent DKA have had continuous hospitalizations of 2 years or more,[12] which would not qualify as brittle diabetes by the 1991 Tattersall definition. Pickup and colleagues emphasized that such severely glycaemically unstable patients were unresponsive to intensified (in their case continuous subcutaneous insulin infusion or CSCII) subcutaneous insulin treatment.[13]

Regardless of these considerations, diabetologists have no difficulty in identifying brittle patients under their care. They defy normal attempts to stabilize their glycaemic instability, have huge hospital case notes and disrupt the life of their diabetes carers as well as their own![1]

Prevalence of brittle diabetes

The estimated frequency of brittle diabetes obviously depends on the definition used. Only one large study has attempted to accurately assess the prevalence of brittle diabetes across a large geographical area. This was a national UK survey carried out in 1995, using the definition 'type 1 diabetes with severe life-disrupting glycaemic instability of any type or cause, associated with recurrent and/or prolonged hospitalisation'.[11] A questionnaire was sent to all UK diabetes clinics, and 414 patients conforming to that definition were reported from an estimated diabetic population of 354 824. Among adult diabetic clinics, the crude prevalence was 0.9 per 1000 patients, amounting to a mean of 1.4 brittle patients per adult diabetic clinic. The prevalence was much higher in paediatric diabetic clinics – 9.8 per 1000, although, because of the smaller size of such clinics, this amounted to a mean of 0.5 brittle patients per paediatric diabetic clinic. Across the whole group, there was a female excess (66%), and the mean age was 26 years. The age distribution of the patients is especially interesting and is shown in Fig. 2.1. It can be seen that

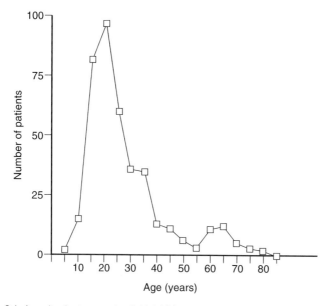

Figure 2.1 *Age distribution graph of 414 UK patients with type 1 diabetes. (From Gill et al[11] with permission.)*

there was a marked peak between 15 and 25 years. Rates declined steeply after the age of 35 years, although there was a small but distinct second peak at age 60–70 years. This phenomenon of 'elderly brittle diabetes' has been previously described,[14–16] and is characterized by more 'mixed' types of glycaemic instability (see next section), and more frequent organic aetiology[17] (see Chapter 9).

The spectrum of glycaemic instability

Most patients with recurrent admissions due to glycaemic instability have stereotyped metabolic patterns – usually either recurrent DKA or recurrent hypoglycaemia. This has been confirmed in three studies – from Nottingham in 1991,[10] Liverpool in 1992[18] (the patients were a combined group from Newcastle and Liverpool) and in a national UK study reported in 1996.[11]

The Nottingham study[10] was of 25 brittle type 1 diabetic patients. 'Recurrent DKA' was defined as three or more admissions with DKA in a 2-year period, and 'recurrent hypoglycaemia' as three or more admissions with severe hypoglycaemia over a similar period. There were 9 (36%) patients with recurrent DKA, a further 9 (36%) with recurrent hypoglycaemia and 7 (28%) with mixed patterns of admissions.

A combined series of Newcastle/Liverpool patients (42 in total) was reported in 1992.[18] It was found that 52% of patients (all female) had recurrent DKA (defined as 90% or more of admissions due to DKA), 24% had 'hyperglycaemic instability' (90% of admissions due to hyperglycaemia, although actual DKA uncommon), 12% had recurrent hypoglycaemia (again, using the '90% or more of admissions' criteria), while 12% had mixed instability with varying admission patterns.

The large national UK study[11] revealed 414 patients with brittle diabetes, and physicians were asked to categorize them as 'recurrent DKA', again using the criteria of 90% or more of admissions being due to DKA. The definition of 'recurrent hypoglycaemia' was similar, and failure to make either of these criteria was termed 'mixed brittle-

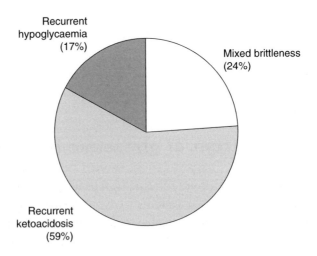

Recurrent hypoglycaemia (17%)

Mixed brittleness (24%)

Recurrent ketoacidosis (59%)

Figure 2.2 *The spectrum of brittle diabetes. Data is from 414 UK brittle type 1 diabetic patients. (From Gill et al[11] with permission.)*

ness'. The proportions were 59% with recurrent DKA, 17% with recurrent hypoglycaemia and 24% with mixed brittleness (see Fig. 2.2).

The study also revealed interesting differences in age and gender characteristics. The recurrent DKA group (59%) had a mean age of 22 years, and there was a marked female excess (male:female ratio 1.0:2.4). Those with recurrent hypoglycaemia (17%) were significantly older with a mean age of 34 years, and the sex ratio was almost equal (male:female 1.0:1.1). The 24% with mixed brittleness were intermediate between the other groups in terms of all parameters studied – mean age 28 years, and male:female ratio 1.0:1.9. Aetiological factors for brittle diabetes will be discussed in the next two sections, but the reasons for these interesting patterns of brittleness have not been adequately explained.

Aetiological factors: organic

As with much in the field of brittle diabetes, there is dispute and controversy over possible aetiologies. This discussion will deal firstly with organic factors and causative disease processes, and then discuss psychological and educational factors. Over the last 10–20 years, there has been general acceptance that the latter group of causes are generally the most common. A summary of the major causes is shown in Table 2.2, and are discussed in more detail below.

Treatment errors
Problems of therapy were quoted extensively as a cause of brittle diabetes in early reviews, but modern insulins and insulin treatment regimens should now make this less likely. However, patient errors should be sought, including injecting into grossly lipohypertrophied areas and also ensuring that the patient is literate, numerate and sighted (attempting to deliver insulin without these skills may be difficult). One form of patient-related glycaemic instability (which in its extreme forms can cause brittle metabolic disturbance) is obsessional self-control.[9,10] These patients have a morbid fear of complications and

Table 2.2 Aetiological factors in brittle diabetes

Organic factors	Psychosocial factors
Treatment errors: most commonly patient-based e.g. compulsive self-control	*Life stress:* with impaired self-treatment decision making
Occult infection: rare and unlikely	*Factitious behaviour:* much recurrent DKA and factitious hypoglycaemia
Alcohol and drug abuse: growing problem	*Eating disorders:* with insulin omission
Endocrine disorders: in particular, hypoadrenalism	*Educational and psycholinguistic disorders:* with disordered information processing and decision making
Gastrointestinal disease: e.g. coeliac disease, diabetic gastropathy	
Subcutaneous insulin resistance: now discredited	
Systemic insulin resistance: e.g. overinsulinisation	

overtreat themselves with insulin, usually causing recurrent hypogly-caemia. Figure 2.3 shows the grossly erratic 'roller-coaster' glycaemic profile of a patient performing 7 or more blood glucose levels per day, and reacting to each one with additional short-acting insulin doses.

Occult infection

This was a commonly invoked cause of brittle diabetes in older reviews, but is rarely experienced in modern clinical practice. In the unusual instance of a type 1 patient developing a significant, chronic and undiagnosed infection, this would generally cause sustained hyperglycaemia rather than recurrent DKA.

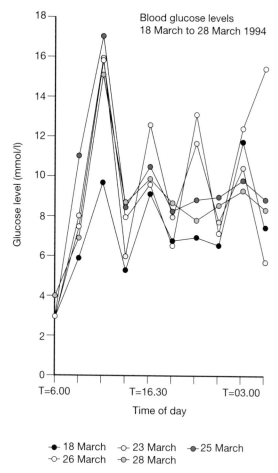

Figure 2.3 *Home blood glucose profiles recorded by a brittle diabetic patient performing several blood glucose tests per day, and reacting to these with soluble insulin boluses, in addition to a twice-daily regimen of a 30/70 soluble/isophane mixture. The graph above was computer-generated by the patient and produced in clinic. The patient had an obsessional desire to be 'well-controlled' (but also serious educational misconceptions!).*

Alcohol and drug abuse

Alcohol abuse has long been known to destabilize type 1 diabetes. Recurrent severe hypoglycaemia may occur, although sometimes chronic poor control or DKA can occur as a result of self-neglect. A more recently described problem concerning drugs and diabetic instability concerns opiate abuse – particularly intravenous cocaine or heroin addiction. These patients may omit insulin, resulting in recurrent DKA. In a US study in 1998, 14% of all DKA admissions were related to cocaine abuse.[19]

Endocrine disorders

Thyrotoxicosis, phaeochromocytoma, acromegaly and Cushing's syndrome may all destabilize existing type 1 diabetes, but do not usually cause brittleness; however, hypoadrenalism (either primary adrenal or secondary to pituitary ACTH deficiency) can greatly increase insulin sensitivity and lead to recurrent and severe hypoglycaemia[20,21] (see Chapter 7).

Gastrointestinal disease

Severe autonomic neuropathy of the bowel can interfere with intestinal transit and carbohydrate absorption. Diabetic gastropathy with recurrent vomiting can particularly destabilize glycaemic control. Coeliac disease (which occurs more frequently in type 1 diabetes) is a well-described cause of hypoglycaemic brittleness.[22]

Subcutaneous insulin resistance

In the early 1980s, it was suggested that some young female type 1 diabetic patients with recurrent DKA, and apparently high subcutaneous insulin requirements, may have a disorder of subcutaneous insulin absorption, as control appeared greatly improved when insulin was delivered by other routes (e.g. intramuscular, intravenous or intraperitoneal).[23] It was suggested that this may be due to impaired subcutaneous blood flow,[24] or increased local protease activity.[25] However, these studies were generally poorly supervised (the importance of patient interference with treatment as a cause of recurrent DKA had not been appreciated at the time). Using very carefully controlled conditions, excluding the possibility of patient interference, Schade and Duckworth in 1986 reported their failure to demonstrate anything but normal insulin absorption in such patients.[26] Few now believe in the existence of subcutaneous insulin resistance (see Chapter 3 for a more detailed discussion of recurrent DKA).

Systemic insulin resistance

There is at least one well-documented report of systemic insulin resistance in a patient with brittle diabetes,[27] as well as other anecdotal reports of intravenous insulin resistance in review articles.[28] It may be that some or all of these occurrences are related to the phenomenon of overinsulinization, sometimes known as Mauriac's syndrome. Here, excessive insulin doses appear to lead to weight gain and poor glycaemic control.[29] Interestingly, there is some evidence that in patients with recurrent DKA, decreased insulin receptor density and reduced sensitivity can be shown,[30] and this down-regulation may improve with resolution of brittleness.[31] This has led to the proposal that even in factitious hyperglycaemic instability, escalating insulin treatment may lead to overinsulinization (such patients are certainly frequently overweight[12,13]), insulin receptor down-regulation and an acquired situation of systemic insulin resistance.[12]

Aetiological factors: psychosocial

Non-organic problems are now well-recognized and are common factors in the genesis of brittle diabetes. These psychosocial factors are complex and diverse (see Table 2.2, and, for a more detailed discussion, Chapter 6).

Life stress

As early as 1949, emotional upset and life stresses were linked to glycaemic instability in type 1 diabetes.[8] This is viewed as a common clinical experience,[9,12,32] but what is less certain is how emotional disturbance may lead to glycaemic instability. Early suggestions of a stress-induced counter-regulatory hormone effect seem unlikely. This could contribute to hyperglycaemic, but not hypoglycaemic or mixed instability. Furthermore, the hyperglycaemic and ketogenic effect of induced hypercatecholaminaemia are modest.[33] An alternative effect may be that life stresses can interfere with the self-management decision-making processes necessary for daily coping with type 1 diabetes.

Factitious behaviour

The seemingly bizarre possibility that some patients deliberately induce either hypoglycaemia or ketoacidosis has been known for some time. Factitious hypoglycaemia has been well described, with reports going back over 50 years.[34] Deliberate induction of DKA as a cause of diabetic brittleness was described particularly in the early 1980s,[12,13,35] although Peck and Peck also described a typical case in 1956.[36] The reason for this self-induced brittleness may be a simple form of escape from intolerable life stresses into the 'safe haven' of hospital (or in the longer-term, into a role of chronic unexplained illness). Not uncommonly, however, there is no obvious reason for this self-destructive behaviour, which occurs in the absence of precipitating life stresses or formal psychiatric disease.[28,37] The term 'medical Munchausen's syndrome' has understandably been used to describe these patients.[20]

Eating disorders

Anorexia nervosa is a psychiatric condition which very understandably may, in combination with type 1 diabetes, lead to insulin dose reduction or omission. Indeed, this is an ideal (if dangerous) method of weight control for the patient unfortunate enough to have such dual pathologies. There is some evidence that eating disorders are over-represented in young females with type 1 diabetes, and that such patients are prone to poor control and episodes of DKA, as well as increased risk of complications.[38,39] Young females with recurrent DKA studied during the early and mid 1980s[12,13,40] (or at least some of them), probably did have eating disorders, and one study from that period identified anorexic 'traits'.[12]

Educational and psycholinguistic disorders

Finally, Schade and colleagues in Albuquerque (New Mexico) identified specific educational deficiencies as a major cause of unstable glycaemic control among their tertiary referrals with brittle diabetes (mostly recurrent DKA).[2,40] Careful evaluation by psychologists and educationalists showed psycholinguistic disorders of information reception and processing that were similar to those found in some individuals with learning disorders. Diabetic control improved following intensive rehabilitation and re-educational treatment.

Natural history

Few studies have examined the natural history of brittle diabetes and most have been focused on recurrent DKA (see Chapter 3). After a mean 10.5 years a 1991 follow-up study from Liverpool of 26 UK patients with severe recurrent DKA showed that 5 (19%) had died, but of the 21 survivors only 2 (10%) were still considered brittle.[41] Microvascular complications were common (67%) and a number had had pregnancy complications. Curiously, 2 of the 5 deaths were due to hypoglycaemia (2 others died from DKA, and 1 in renal failure).

Williams and Pickup in 1988 reported a 3–6 year follow-up of 13 patients with brittle diabetes:[42] 5 of the group had recurrent DKA, 1 recurrent hypoglycaemia and 7 mixed instability. During the relatively short follow-up period, there was one death – again from hypoglycaemia (she was one of the patients with recurrent DKA). Brittleness improved in the survivors, but only one patient was considered metabolically stable.

Finally, a 1991 Nottingham study reported 25 brittle patients with varying types of instability followed for 12 years.[10] There were 5 deaths – 2 from renal failure, 2 from hypoglycaemia, and 1 unrelated to diabetes (cerebral tumour). Most patients tended to show improved control during follow-up.

In all of these studies brittle diabetes appeared to be closely related to life stresses and psychosocial problems, whereas resolution of brittleness corresponded often to positive life events. For example, one consultant in the Liverpool study,[41] commented that his patient (now stable): 'seemed to have settled into an uneventful life following her marriage; she has not been admitted for some years now and at one stage was in every fortnight'.

Despite this tendency to resolution, brittle diabetes is clearly shown by these studies to be associated with significant morbidity and premature mortality. Of the 64 patients in the three studies reviewed above, 11 died (17%). Almost half of these deaths (5) were due to hypoglycaemia – perhaps, surprisingly, as most cases had hyperglycaemic instability. Interestingly, 2 patients have been described with hyperglycaemic brittle diabetes who later developed recurrent hypoglycaemia – 1 patient due to the development of Addison's disease[43] and 1 patient due to the factitious administration of insulin.[44]

Assessment and investigation

Newly presenting or referred patients with brittle diabetes should be evaluated efficiently and rapidly. Protracted and indecisive investigation often becomes counterproductive and demanding for both patient and doctor. Clinical algorithms for brittle diabetes investigation have been proposed,[32,45] but these are not always easily applicable to complex individual cases, and it may be more appropriate to individualize the assessment process.

Figure 2.4 shows that assessment strategies depend to some extent on the pattern of glycaemic instability. Organic causes are more likely to be found in recurrent hypoglycaemia, and investigations such as autonomic function tests, antigliadin antibodies (for possible coeliac disease) and a Short Synacthen Test (to exclude hypoadrenalism) may be indicated. If organic causes cannot be found, factitious hypoglycaemia should be considered,[34] and C-peptide levels during hypoglycaemic episodes (or possibly a 'locker search' for hidden insulin supplies) may be needed.[12,46]

By contrast, most recurrent DKA is behavioural in origin, and life 'chaos' or crises should be sought, as well as possible anorexic syndromes[47] and psycholinguistic and/or educational disorders.[40] Factitiously induced DKA due to insulin reduction or omission is relatively

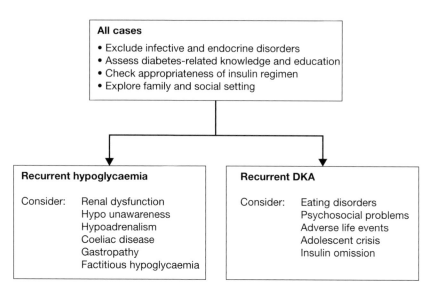

All cases

- Exclude infective and endocrine disorders
- Assess diabetes-related knowledge and education
- Check appropriateness of insulin regimen
- Explore family and social setting

Recurrent hypoglycaemia

Consider: Renal dysfunction
               Hypo unawareness
               Hypoadrenalism
               Coeliac disease
               Gastropathy
               Factitious hypoglycaemia

Recurrent DKA

Consider: Eating disorders
               Psychosocial problems
               Adverse life events
               Adolescent crisis
               Insulin omission

Figure 2.4 *Assessment of the patient with brittle diabetes. Note that in patients with mixed glycaemic instability, investigation should be individualized and may include investigations as above for both recurrent DKA and hypoglycaemic brittleness.*

common.[48] Such patients often have apparent insulin resistance (high subcutaneous insulin doses but poor glycaemic control), and Schade and colleagues in the United States have described techniques for demonstrating normal insulin absorption and requirements. These include ward cubicle 'imprisonment' tactics to exclude interference with or omission of insulin treatment, or a carefully controlled subcutaneous insulin absorption test[2,26,37,40] (see Chapter 5).

Management strategies

The specific management of recurrent DKA and recurrent hypoglycaemia are covered in detail in Chapters 3 and 7, respectively. The four management strategies for brittle diabetes are outlined in Table 2.3 and are discussed in detail below.

Table 2.3 Management strategies for brittle diabetes

1. *Potentially curative:*
   Hypoadrenalism
   Coeliac disease
   Eating disorders
2. *Psychological:*
   Structured support
   Psychotherapy
   Cognitive analytical therapy (CAT)
3. *Life-preserving:*
   Continuous intraperitoneal insulin infusion (CIPII)
   Implantable insulin pump
   Pancreas transplantation
4. *Expectant:*
   Most brittle diabetes resolves with time

Potentially curative

Few patients have underlying causes which are correctable. Examples include hydrocortisone replacement in Addison's disease, dietary exclusion of gluten in coeliac disease and successful psychologically based treatment of anorexia nervosa.

Psychological

Where no organic cause is found after appropriate investigation, it is reasonable to conclude that brittleness is non-organic and related to psychological or social problems. In such cases, it is logical to aim treatment primarily at these factors, rather than to adopt a blind 'mechanistic' approach (e.g. insulin pumps etc. – see below). Formal psychiatric disease is rarely present, and psychiatric referral is usually non-productive.[12] However, clinical psychologists (especially those with an interest and experience in diabetes care) may be valuable, both in assessment and treatment. Psychotherapeutic treatment can be helpful,[49] notably cognitive analytical therapy (CAT),[50] although psychologists with experience of both CAT and brittle diabetes are scarce. Simple supportive care and counselling from members of the diabetes team can be effective, but the patient should be encouraged to be independent rather than dependent: one patient, for example, with very severe recurrent hypoglycaemia broke out of their cycle of admissions following structured support from a community social worker.[51]

Life-preserving

Previously described treatments for refractory brittle diabetes have included addition of aprotinin or prostaglandins to insulin, plasmapheresis, haemodialysis and various non-subcutaneous routes of insulin delivery (intramuscular, intravenous and intraperitoneal).[32] These highly 'mechanistic' approaches should be avoided if possible,[52] as the treatments either do not work or have potentially hazardous complications. An expectant policy is to be preferred if possible (see below). However, some severely brittle diabetic patients with recurrent DKA develop a serious lack of peripheral, and sometimes even central veins,[12] and here the syndrome can become life-threatening. In this situation 'rescue' intervention to preserve life may be reasonable, in an attempt to 'buy time' until natural resolution of brittleness hopefully occurs. Treatments reported to be successful in this situation include continuous intraperitoneal insulin infusion (CIPII),[53] continuous intravenous or intraperitoneal infusion by fully implantable ('Infusaid') pumps[54] and even pancreatic transplantation[55] (see Chapter 13).

Expectant

If the situation is not life-threatening, a policy of 'masterly inactivity' may be reasonable. The rationale is that most brittle diabetes resolves with time, and that over-mechanistic treatments allow further hospital dependence and give elevated patient status, and are prone to significant side effects. The counter-argument is of course that prolonged brittleness is associated with an increased complication and mortality risk long term.[41]

Conclusions

Brittle diabetes is best regarded as the extreme end of a spectrum of disordered glycaemic control related to adverse life events and/or maladaptation to chronic disease. Studies on HbA_{1c} levels in large numbers of 'non-brittle' diabetic patients have shown that levels are higher in females than in males,[56] younger compared with older,[57] and in those with family stresses.[58] These characteristics are shared with subjects who have clinically obvious brittle diabetes.

Diabetes is also not the only chronic disease to have its uncontrollable minority. Interestingly, 'brittle asthma'[59] and 'brittle Addison's disease'[60] have been described, and most such patients are young and female.

Brittle diabetes is thus a complex mixture of the organic and the functional, particularly affecting those with adverse life stresses, psychosocial disturbances or an uneasy relationship with their condition. The type 1 diabetic patient with refractory brittleness of any type still presents the diabetes care team with one of the most daunting challenges in clinical diabetology.

References

1. Gill GV. Does brittle diabetes exist? In: Gill GV, Pickup JC, Williams G, eds, Difficult diabetes. Blackwell Science, Oxford, 2000: 151–67.
2. Schade DS. Brittle diabetes – strategies, diagnosis and treatment. Diab Metab Rev 1988; 4: 371–90.
3. Williams G, Gill GV, Pickup JC. Brittle diabetes. Br Med J 1991; 303: 714.
4. Tattersall RB. Brittle diabetes revisited – the 3rd Arnold Bloom Memorial Lecture. Diabet Med 1997; 14: 94–110.
5. Haunz EA. An approach to the problem of the brittle diabetic patient: a study of 6 cases. JAMA 1950; 142: 168–73.
6. Wilder RM. Clinical diabetes and hyperinsulinism. WB Saunders, Philadelphia, 1940: 100–1.
7. Molnar GD. Observations on the aetiology and therapy of 'brittle' diabetes. Canad Med Assoc J 1964; 90: 953–9.

8. Rosen H, Lidz T. Emotional factors in the precipitation of recurrent diabetic acidosis. Psychosom Med 1949; 11: 211–15.
9. Tattersall R. Brittle diabetes. Clin Endocrinol Metab 1977; 6: 403–19.
10. Tattersall R, Gregory R, Selby C, Kerr D, Heller S. Course of brittle diabetes: a 12 year follow-up. Br Med J 1991; 302: 1240–3.
11. Gill GV, Lucas S, Kent LA. Prevalence and characteristics of brittle diabetes in Britain. Quart J Med 1996; 89: 839–43.
12. Gill GV, Husband DJ, Walford S et al. Clinical features of brittle diabetes. In: Pickup JC, ed, Brittle diabetes. Blackwell Science, Oxford, 1985: 29–40.
13. Pickup JC, Williams G, Johns P, Keen H. Clinical features of brittle diabetic patients unresponsive to optimised subcutaneous insulin therapy (continuous subcutaneous insulin infusion). Diabetes Care 1983; 6: 279–84
14. Gale EAM, Dornan TL, Tattersall RB. Severe untreated diabetes in the over-fifties. Diabetologia 1981; 21: 25–8.
15. Chapman J, Wright AD, Nattrass M, Fitzgerald MG. Recurrent diabetic ketoacidosis. Diabet Med 1988; 5: 659–81.
16. Griffith DNW, Yudkin JS. Brittle diabetes in the elderly. Diabet Med 1989; 6: 400–43.
17. Benbow S, Walsh A, Gill GV. Brittle diabetes in the elderly – a UK study. J Roy Soc Med 2001; 94: 578–80.
18. Gill GV. The spectrum of brittle diabetes. J Roy Soc Med 1992; 85: 259–61.
19. Warner EA, Greene GS, Buchsbaum MS, Cooper DS, Robinson BE. Diabetic ketoacidosis with cocaine use. Arch Int Med 1998; 158: 1799–802.
20. Gale EAM, Tattersall R. Brittle diabetes. Br J Hosp Med 1979; 21: 589–97.
21. Hardy KJ, Burge MR, Boyle PJ, Scarpello JHB. A treatable cause of recurrent severe hypoglycaemia. Diabetes Care 1994; 17: 722–4.
22. Bhattacharyya A, Tymms DJ. Life-threatening hypoglycaemia due to previously unrecognised coeliac disease in a patient with type 1 diabetes mellitus. Pract Diabetes Int 1999; 16: 90–2.
23. Pickup JC, Home PD, Bilous RW, Alberti KGMM, Keen H. Management of severely brittle diabetes by continuous subcutaneous and intramuscular insulin infusion: evidence for a defect in subcutaneous insulin absorption. Br Med J 1981; 282: 347–50.
24. Williams G, Pickup JC, Clark AJL et al. Changes in blood flow due to subcutaneous insulin injection sites in stable and brittle diabetics. Diabetes 1983; 32: 466–73.
25. Friedenberg GR, White N, Cataland S et al. Diabetes responsive to intravenous but not subcutaneous insulin: effectiveness of aprotonin. N Engl J Med 1981; 305: 363–8.
26. Schade DS, Duckworth WC. In search of the subcutaneous insulin resistance syndrome. N Engl J Med 1986; 315: 147–53.

27. Williams G, Pickup JC, Keen H. Massive insulin resistance apparently due to rapid clearance of circulating insulin. Am J Med 1987; 82: 1247–52.

28. Gill GV, Walford S, Alberti KGMM. Brittle diabetes – present concepts. Diabetologia 1985; 28: 579–89.

29. Rosenbloom AL, Giordano BP. Chronic overtreatment with insulin in children and adolescents. Am J Dis Childhood 1977; 131: 881–5.

30. Taylor R, Husband DJ, Marshall SM, Tunbridge WMG, Alberti KGMM. Adipocyte insulin binding and insulin sensitivity in 'brittle' diabetes. Diabetologia 1984; 27: 441–6.

31. Taylor R, Hetherington CS, Gill GV, Alberti KGMM. Changes in tissue insulin sensitivity in previously 'brittle' diabetes. Horm Metab Res 1986; 18: 493.

32. Gill GV, Williams G. Causes and management of poor metabolic control. In: Pickup JC, Williams G, eds, Textbook of diabetes, 3rd edn. Blackwell Science, Oxford, 2002: 43.21–38.

33. Pernet A, Walker M, Gill GV et al. Metabolic effects of adrenaline and noradrenaline in man: studies with somatostatin. Diabet Metab 1984; 10: 98–105.

34. Orr DP, Eccles T, Lawler R, Golden M. Surreptitious insulin administration in adolescents with insulin dependent diabetes mellitus. JAMA 1986; 256: 3227–30.

35. Flexnor CW, Weiner JP, Saudek CD, Dans PF. Repeated hospitalisations for diabetic ketoacidosis. The game of 'Sartoris'. Am J Med 1984; 76: 691–5.

36. Peck FB, Peck FB. Tautologous diabetic coma – a behaviour syndrome. Multiple unnecessary episodes of diabetic coma. Diabetes 1956; 5: 44–6.

37. Schade DS, Drumm DA, Eaton RP, Sterling WA. Factitious brittle diabetes. Am J Med 1985; 78: 777–84.

38. Steel JM, Young RJ, Lloyd GG, Clarke BF. Clinically apparent eating disorders in young diabetic women associated with painful neuropathy and other complications. Br Med J 1987; 284: 859–62.

39. Stancin T, Link DL, Reuter JM. Binge eating and purging in young women with IDDM. Diabetes Care 1989; 12: 601–3.

40. Schade DS, Drumm DA, Duckworth WC, Eaton P. The etiology of incapacitating brittle diabetes. Diabetes Care 1985; 8: 12–20.

41. Kent LA, Gill GV, Williams G. Mortality and outcome of patients with brittle diabetes and recurrent ketoacidosis. Lancet 1994; 344: 778–81.

42. Williams G, Pickup JC. The natural history of brittle diabetes. Diabetes Res 1988; 7: 13–18.

43. Naing K, Wijenaike N, Green F, Leese GP, Newton RW. Recurrent hypoglycaemia in a patient with history of brittle diabetes. Pract Diabetes Int 2001; 18: 13–15.

44. Gill GV, Kent L, Williams G, Walford S, Alberti KGMM. An unusual case of relapsing brittle diabetes. Pract Diabetes 1995; 12: 38–9.

45. Schade DS, Eaton P, Drumm DA, Duckworth WC. A clinical algorithm to determine the etiology of brittle diabetes. Diabetes Care 1985; 8: 5–11.

46. Scarlett JA, Mako ME, Rubenstein AH et al. Factitious hypoglycaemia: Diagnosis by measurement of serum C-peptide immunoreactivity and insulin binding antibodies. N Engl J Med 1977; 297: 1029–32.

47. Jones JM, Lawson ML, Daneman D, Olmsted MP, Rodin G. Eating disorders in adolescent females with and without type 1 diabetes: cross-sectional study. Br Med J 2000; 320: 1563–6.

48. Polonsky WH, Aponte JE, Anderson BJ et al. Insulin omission in women with IDDM. Diabetes Care 1994; 17: 1178–85.

49. Moran G, Fonagy P, Kurtz A, Bolton A, Brook C. A controlled study of the psychoanalytic treatment of brittle diabetes. J Am Acad Child Adolesc Psychiat 1991; 30: 926–35.

50. Ryle A, Boa C, Fosbury J. Identifying the causes of poor self-management in insulin-dependent diabetes: the use of cognitive-analytical therapy techniques. In: Hodes M, Mooney S, eds, Psychological treatment in disease and illness. Gaskell/Society for Psychosomatic Research, London, 1993: 157–65.

51. Gill GV, Robinson M, Marrow J. Hypoglycaemic brittle diabetes successfully managed by social worker intervention. Diabetic Med 1989; 6: 448–50.

52. Gill GV. Brittle diabetes. Current Medical Literature – Diabetes 1990; 7: 31–5.

53. DeVries JH, Eskes SA, Snoek FJ et al. Continuous intraperitoneal insulin infusion in patients with 'brittle' diabetes: favourable effects on glycaemic control and hospital stay. Diabet Med 2002; 19: 496–501.

54. Gill GV, Husband DJ, Wright PD et al. The management of severe brittle diabetes with 'Infusaid' implantable pumps. Diabetes Res 1986; 3: 135–7.

55. Robinson ACP, Pacy P, Kearney T et al. Pancreatic transplantation in 'brittle diabetes mellitus' – a case report. Diabet Med 1996; 13(Suppl 7): S11.

56. Strickland MII, Patam RC, Wales JK. Haemoglobin A1c concentrations in men and women with diabetes. Br Med J 1984; 289: 753.

57. Pound N, Sturrock NDC, Jeffcoate WJ. Age-related changes in glycated haemoglobin in patients with insulin-dependent diabetes mellitus. Diabet Med 1996; 13: 510–13.

58. Vince R, McGrath M, Trudinger P. Family stress and metabolic control in diabetes. Arch Dis Childhood 1996; 74: 418–22.

59. Ayres JG, Miles JF, Barnes PJ. Brittle asthma. Thorax 1998; 53: 315–21.

60. Gill GV, Williams G. Brittle Addison's disease: a new variation on a familiar theme. Postgrad Med J 2000; 76: 166–7.

chapter 3

The syndrome of recurrent diabetic ketoacidosis

Geoff Gill and George Alberti

Introduction

One of the best-recognized patterns of glycaemic instability in severely unstable or 'brittle' type 1 diabetes is the syndrome of recurrent diabetic ketoacidosis (DKA). These patients contribute about two-thirds of the total burden of brittle diabetes, and are almost always young (in their teens and twenties) and female.[1,2] They have recurrent admissions with DKA, which persist despite all therapeutic interventions, and, not surprisingly, they have significant mortality and an increased later burden of diabetic complications. Their 'brittleness', however, may resolve with the passage of time, and they can resume acceptable glycaemic stability.[3] This chapter will trace the history of the syndrome of recurrent DKA, critically examine causative theories, and review management and outcome.

Birth of a syndrome – 1949 to 1956

Although recurrent DKA in type 1 diabetes was largely described and investigated in the late 1970s and early 1980s, a number of overlooked

American reports 30 years previously accurately recorded the same condition. In 1949, Hinkle and Wolf described a 15-year-old girl who had been hospitalized 14 times with DKA since her original diagnosis 4 years previously.[4] She was obese and emotionally disturbed, and close observations by the authors led them to conclude that her episodes of DKA were related to family upsets, and perhaps mediated by stress hormone secretion. Later the same year, Rosen and Lidz reported a series of 12 patients with type 1 diabetes with a mean occurrence rate of 5.5 attacks of DKA per patient (2 had more than 15 episodes).[5] Details of age and gender were not given, but from some of the case descriptions given in the paper, it appears the group were of mixed gender and various ages. Emotional disturbances were again thought to be aetiologically important, as well as in some cases omission of insulin (occasionally suicidal).

In 1952, Hinkle and Wolf described a series of observations on type 1 diabetic patients demonstrating a close relationship between emotional stress and glycaemic control.[6] One of these patients was a 15-year-old schoolgirl who had been 'referred to the diabetic clinic because of recurrent episodes of ketonuria, which had continued despite all efforts to abolish them by changes in diet or insulin intake.' She came from a high-achieving professional family (her father and brother were doctors) who forced her into academic work and curtailed her social life. The authors reported some improvement in her diabetic control following what amounted to family psychotherapy.

Finally, in 1956 Peck and Peck reported the case of a 20-year-old female type 1 diabetic patient, who had experienced at least 42 episodes of DKA since diagnosis at age 12 years.[7] The patient had severe psychosocial problems, coming from a broken home with a criminal mother and alcoholic father. Many of the attacks of DKA were life threatening, and the authors believed at least some to be due to insulin omission – 'an unpleasant stressful situation was met habitually by precipitation of a bout of acidosis and coma and removal from the life stress to the more sympathetic hospital environment.'

Rediscovery of a syndrome – 1979 to 1984

Although further cases must have occurred, no more was heard of the syndrome of recurrent DKA until the late 1970s. In two review articles on brittle diabetes from Nottingham[8,9] in 1977 and 1979, respectively, the 'emotional causes' of brittle diabetes were reviewed, including reference to the early papers by Rosen and Lidz,[5] and Peck and Peck.[7] Glycaemic instability by 'deliberate manipulation' was also discussed, and even the term 'medical Munchausen's syndrome' was used.

Around the time of these reports, and in the ensuing 8 years, patients with severe and marked recurrent DKA began to present, and were investigated in detail in two centres in the UK (Newcastle-upon-Tyne and London) and three in the USA (Baltimore, New York and New Mexico). These groups reported their experiences between 1983 and 1985.[10–15] The Newcastle series was of 19 patients who had collectively experienced a remarkable 410 episodes of DKA.[10,11] Their hospitalizations were not only frequent, but often also prolonged (in one case over 2 years). All the patients were female, and their mean age was 19 years.

The London group[12] was of 14 unstable type 1 patients, 12 of whom had recurrent DKA. They were all female, with ages ranging from 13 to 27 years. Many were overweight, and the authors suggested a relationship between the age of onset of brittleness and the age of menarche. As well as recurrent admissions with DKA, the patients were uncontrollable on optimized insulin regimes, including continuous subcutaneous insulin infusion (CSII).

In 1984, Flexner and colleagues from Baltimore, USA, reported a group of 45 type 1 diabetic patients with recurrent DKA.[13] Their definition of recurrent DKA was relatively loose (over 2 admissions with DKA in a 30-month period), but nevertheless many patients clearly were similar to those reported from Newcastle and London in the UK. Detailed case histories were recorded of 3 patients with a mean 11 admissions annually with DKA. The authors believed that in the majority of cases, DKA was caused by 'therapeutic recidivism', and poor compliance with therapy was frequently suspected.

In 1985, Fulop in New York reported 17 patients who were 'hospitalized repeatedly for diabetic ketoacidosis' (a group total of 92 episodes).[14] The patients were of mixed sex, but females were greatly over-represented in those with particularly large numbers of admissions. Most patients were young. No particular comments or conclusions were made as to the cause of DKA recurrence, although poor compliance was suspected in 6 patients.

Finally, in 1985, Schade and colleagues[15,16] reported on 30 type 1 diabetic patients, referred to their centre in Albuquerque, New Mexico, USA. Twenty-three were female, and most patients were in their twenties and overweight. Factitious causes of instability were regarded as present in about one-half of the group; and other causes included 'communication disorders' and 'insulin resistance' (both of which will be discussed in detail later). Although many of these patients had recurrent DKA, some had recurrent hypoglycaemic episodes.

Characteristics of patients with recurrent DKA

The reports referred to above from the UK and USA,[10–15] as well as earlier studies from the late 1940s, and early 1950s,[4–7] provide a remarkably stereotyped picture. Quantitative details of the characteristics of the Newcastle group of 19 patients[10] are shown in Table 3.1, but the major features are as follows:

- young age
- female sex
- multiple episodes of DKA
- recurrent and/or prolonged admissions
- overweight
- therapeutic control failure
- high insulin doses.

The term 'control failure' alludes to the fact that these patients could not achieve any semblance of control on standard (twice-daily

Table 3.1 Clinical features of 19 patients with the syndrome of recurrent DKA, studied in Newcastle, UK (means ± SEM)[10]

Number	19
Age (years)	18.3 ± 0.9 (range 13–27)
Sex	All female
Duration diabetes (years)	8.0 ± 1.0 (range 2–18)
Duration brittle (years)	2.2 ± 0.4 (range 1–8)
Daily insulin dose (units)	144 ± 14 (range 30–232)
Percentage ideal body weight	120 ± 3 (range 107–152)
Episodes of DKA	Total 410 for whole group (zero mortality)

soluble/isophane insulin mixtures subcutaneously), or intensified (multiple dose subcutaneous insulin or CSII) insulin systems.[12] Perhaps because of this problem, they tended to be on high and escalating insulin doses, although glycaemic control remained poor with high HbA$_{1c}$ levels.

Recurrent DKA makes up the largest subgroup of patients with brittle diabetes (59% of all brittle patients in a UK survey), with recurrent hypoglycaemia (17%) and 'mixed brittleness' (24%) making up the rest.[2]

Causative theories of recurrent DKA

Two major opposing concepts of the causation of recurrent DKA have emerged – not surprisingly representing the functional and the organic. However, there are two other later-proposed theories that are of interest. The early reports in the late 1940s and early 1950s saw the condition as predominantly emotionally based, but were uncertain whether DKA resulted from interference with therapy, or was due to a hormonally-mediated stress response. By the late 1970s, however, diabetology was increasingly scientifically based, and an organic cause for the syndrome of recurrent DKA was hotly pursued. The four proposed theories will therefore be considered in approximate chronological order, between 1979 and 1985.

Subcutaneous insulin resistance?

The most celebrated, and apparently plausible, pathophysiological explanation for recurrent DKA was that of 'subcutaneous insulin resistance'. This was first proposed by Dandona and colleagues, from London, in 1978.[17] These workers described 6 patients with unstable type 1 diabetes who required several hundred units of subcutaneous insulin daily, but only 50–60 units intravenously. A combined report from the London and Newcastle groups in 1981 demonstrated similarly improved control on smaller doses of insulin by using the intramuscular rather than the subcutaneous route, demonstrating 'evidence for a defect in subcutaneous insulin absorption'.[18] The nature of this 'absorption defect' was investigated by a variety of techniques, including decay curves of injected radio-labelled insulin, subcutaneous haemodynamic studies and enzymic studies on biopsy tissue samples. Results were somewhat inconsistent, but evidence was presented for increased enzymic degradation of insulin at subcutaneous injection sites,[19] and also for reduced subcutaneous blood flow[20] – both processes supposedly reducing insulin effectiveness when delivered subcutaneously, but allowing normal activity by other routes.

Pure factitious instability?

In 1984[21] and 1985,[10] however, evidence was presented by the Newcastle group that deliberate interference with therapy may be the major causation of recurrent DKA. In a group of 19 young females (mean age 18 years) with brittle type 1 diabetes, and a mean number of DKA episodes of 22 per year, Gill and colleagues found evidence of self-induction of DKA in 10 patients (53%).[10,21] There were strong suspicions of similar factitious behaviour in the others. Simple cessation of insulin injections was frequent, but for those on insulin infusion treatment, more sinister manipulative behaviour occurred. This included damage to pumps and infusion lines, and also dilution of insulin solutions in intravenous infusion devices. Tap water was often used, sometimes resulting in unusual septicaemic episodes. In one Newcastle patient this was detected by abnormally low sodium levels in the pump fluid (which should have been 0.9% saline with insulin). Amazingly, this patient then learnt to dilute her pump fluid with sterile 0.9% saline ampoules (stolen from the ward drug trolley) – resulting in further DKA episodes but normal sodium levels in the pump fluid! Soon after these observations, in 1986, Schade and Duckworth in the USA reported similar experiences. They had studied 16 young female type 1 diabetic patients referred from various parts of the USA.[22] All had recurrent DKA and a diagnosis of 'subcutaneous insulin resistance'. Using 'imprisonment tactics' (i.e. continuous observation and total supervision of insulin administration), all patients became entirely controllable from a glycaemic viewpoint. Standard subcutaneous insulin challenges were also performed (0.1 units/kg, again under controlled situations with fresh insulin) and blood glucose dropped appropriately. By the mid and late 1980s, the causative pendulum had swung away from an organic cause for recurrent DKA (in particular 'subcutaneous malabsorption'), and the evidence appeared firmly in favour of a behavioural aetiology.

A combined functional/organic theory

Although the concept of subcutaneous malabsorption was discredited, other metabolic abnormalities in patients with recurrent DKA remained unexplained. These included hyperlactataemia,[23] occasional clearly documented massive intravenous insulin resistance,[24] and an exaggerated glycaemic and ketonaemic response to insulin withdrawal.[25] The latter experiments were particularly carefully controlled and supervised, and showed significantly higher blood glucose and plasma ketone responses to the cessation of intravenous insulin in recurrent DKA patients, compared with a group of stable type 1 patients. In addition, the evidence for a completely factitious

47

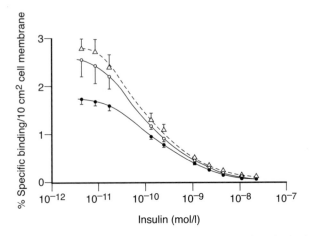

Figure 3.1 *Graph showing specific insulin binding to adipocytes from brittle diabetic patients with recurrent DKA (n = 6, filled circles), 'stable' type 1 diabetic patients (n = 7, open circles), and normal control subjects (n = 6, triangles). The brittle patients show significantly reduced insulin receptor binding. (Reproduced from reference 26 with permission.)*

aetiology is incomplete. Deliberate manipulation of therapy was only proved in just over half of patients.[21] Some patients with recurrent DKA also reported that although they had initially induced deliberate metabolic decompensation, later they developed genuine instability despite attempts at therapeutic compliance.[10] A clue to resolving these ideas may lie in insulin receptor sensitivity. Elegant studies by Taylor and colleagues of the Newcastle group showed reduced adipocyte insulin receptor affinity in a group of recurrent DKA patients[26] (Figure 3.1). It was later shown in 3 of these patients that when brittleness later resolved, these markers of insulin resistance improved.[27] This suggests that the patients were 'overinsulinized', and accords with the consistent finding of their being overweight (which is the reverse of what would be expected in purely insulin-deficient states). These observations led the Newcastle group to propose a 'vicious circle' theory of the genesis and maintenance of brittle diabetes due to recurrent DKA[10,28] (Figure 3.2). Here it is suggested that initially self-induced hyperglycaemia and DKA is responded to by iatrogenic

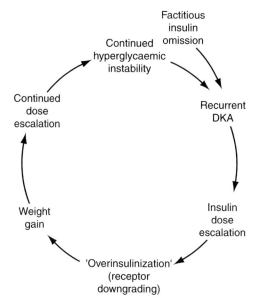

Figure 3.2 *The 'vicious circle' hypothesis of how initially self-induced DKA can be maintained. (From reference 28 with permission.)*

insulin dose escalation, leading to 'overinsulinization' with receptor downgrading and an acquired insulin resistance situation leading to continued hyperglycaemic instability despite self-attempts at therapeutic compliance.

A psycholinguistic disorder

A radically different explanation for severe brittleness in type 1 diabetes was suggested by Schade and colleagues from New Mexico, again in the mid 1980s.[15,16,29] Using detailed evaluation by psychologists and speech therapists, these workers reported psycholinguistic communicative disorders in some patients, whereby central cerebral information processing was disordered although sensory input was intact (e.g. vision, hearing, etc.). Thus, diabetes-related education and therapy-related instructions may not be translated into correct decisions on self-care.[30] Psycholinguistic disorders are well-recognized in the field of both childhood and adult learning disorders,[31] but had not been previously described in unstable diabetes. The US group found evidence of some form of communicative disorder in 7 of a series of 30 brittle diabetic patients (23%),[15] many of whom showed clinical improvement with psychological and educational therapy.

An aetiological overview

It can be appreciated that reports and research on patients with recurrent DKA have shown a rather strange circle of aetiological theories – starting with psychological, moving to organic, and later returning to psychological (as well as perhaps educational). Indeed, the early reports of patients with recurrent DKA (from 1949 to 1956) did not entirely agree on causation. Rosen and Lidz (1949) believed their patients suffered DKA because of 'abandonment of their regime',[5] and Peck and Peck (1956) also reported their single patient to have induced repeated attacks of DKA to avoid family-related stress[7] (their paper was entitled 'Tautologous diabetic coma – a behaviour syndrome'). Hinkle and Wolf, however,[4,6] suggested that psychosocial stress led to metabolic decompensation via counter-regulatory hormone secretion. Although still a widely believed effect, the evidence for such a link is poor. Both standardized psychological stress tests in type 1 diabetes,[32] and induced hypercatecholaminaemia in insulin-deficient man,[33] have only mild hyperglycaemic effects. It seems likely, therefore, that adverse psychosocial events and/or 'life chaos' induce destabilization by the patient opting to directly interfere with treatment as an escape mechanism, or possibly by subconscious interference with self-treatment decisions[28] (possibly analogous here to the psycholinguistic communication disorders proposed by Schade and colleagues as of causative importance in at least some patients[15,16,29]).

Although therapeutic manipulation is common in recurrent DKA, it is by no means always possible to identify a life stress from which the subject needs to escape. In this respect, Schade et al differentiate 'malingering' (where there is a reason for induction of DKA) from factitious behaviour (where there is not).[15,16,29] The classical 'factitious' patient is a 'nice girl' with a 'nice family'.[34] Rosen and Lidz called their patients 'self-destructive',[5] and Gale and Tattersall described the behaviour as 'sheer fecklessness'.[9] An American paper by Flexner and colleagues in 1984,[13] termed the whole meaningless but dangerous scenario 'The game of Sartoris' after a 1929 novel by William Faulkner. The book described the decline and self-destructive demise of a family in the southern USA ('a glamorous fatality').[35]

In an attempt to probe more deeply into the psychopathology of recurrent DKA, Gill and colleagues subjected their patients from Newcastle, UK, to formal psychiatric and psychological evaluation.[10,21] Of their 19 patients, 8 were seen by a psychiatrist and 11 by a psychologist. No psychiatric abnormalities were found, but the psychologist noted an unusual serenity and *belle indifference* to their serious medical plight. Psychometric evaluation revealed a stereotyped pattern of low self-sufficiency and high group-dependency (interestingly, 36 years previously Rosen and Lidz had observed a 'longing for dependency' in their patients[5]).

Table 3.2 reviews qualitative experience from the research reviewed above – the series of quotations perhaps gives something of an insight

Table 3.2 The patient with self-induced recurrent DKA: building a picture from qualitative experience

'self-destructive'	Rosen and Lidz, 1949[5]
'sheer fecklessness'	Gale and Tattersall, 1979[9]
'metabolic Munchausen's syndrome'	Gale and Tattersall, 1979[9]
'such a nice girl'	Steel, 1994[34]
'a Mr Micawber-like optimism'	Gill et al, 1985[10]
'a glamorous fatality'	Flexner and Weiner, 1984[13]
'a serenity and optimism at odds with their predicament'	Gill et al, 1984[21]

into the strange behaviour pattern of the patient with self-induced recurrent DKA. Some insights into this behaviour exist outside the field of diabetes. Recurrent DKA patients are almost exclusively young females, and this marked age and gender characteristic is reminiscent of syndromes of 'female habitual self-mutilation' in general,[36] and anorexia nervosa in particular (indeed, a number of patients with recurrent DKA have been identified as having eating disorders[37]). Joseph has described an 'addiction to near death',[38] and in this respect it is interesting that despite enormous numbers of DKA events in these patients, mortality in ketoacidosis is negligible (no deaths in 410 episodes of DKA in one series[10]). It may be that the 'Game of Sartoris' involves a pattern of behaviour in which life is led 'in the fast lane'; possibly an extreme form of adolescent rebellion (as Naish has remarked, in relation to anorexia nervosa: 'Watch me, mum, I can dice with death and there isn't a thing you can do about it'[39]). Interestingly, both brittle asthma[40] and brittle Addison's disease[41] have been described – again involving young females predominantly, and with evidence of compliance failures.[41] It may be that psychosocial and cultural factors put young females at a disadvantage in adapting to and coping with chronic disease requiring significant elements of self-care[28] (the so-called 'fragile female diabetic'[42]).

None of the discussion above excludes occasional other possibilities of causation, as discussed in the preceding section; but they are probably rare. 'Subcutaneous insulin resistance' has been essentially discredited as a diagnosis,[22] and it is now known that in earlier studies suggestive of such an effect,[18,19] the patients either did not receive prescribed subcutaneous insulin, took greatly reduced doses or used vials of insulin which had been diluted. Nevertheless, even under carefully controlled circumstances, genuine insulin resistance has been recorded by the London,[24,43] Newcastle[11,28,43] and Albuquerque[15,16,29] groups. These few patients have had intravenous (i.e. systemic) rather that subcutaneous insulin resistance, and in at least some cases brittleness has later resolved, with a return to more usual doses of subcutaneous insulin.[3] This is supportive evidence for the 'vicious circle' theory referred to earlier, suggesting that these patients became overinsulinized with receptor downgrading and a secondary systemic insulin resistance.[10,26,27]

Natural history and outcome

There are relatively few studies examining the long-term outcome of patients with brittle diabetes. Some are of mixed cohorts (i.e. not all patients had recurrent DKA) – for example, reports of groups studied in Nottingham[44] and London.[45] A cohort from Newcastle with recurrent DKA only were, however, followed to a mean 8 years after presentation.[46] Most importantly, a large combined group (Newcastle and London) of 33 patients with the syndrome of recurrent DKA were examined in detail at a mean 10 years after original assessment, and compared with a 'stable' control group[3].

The Nottingham study[44] was of 25 patients with varying types of glycaemic instability, 11 of whom had recurrent DKA. The definition was relatively conservative – 3 or more DKA admissions in a 2-year period. Interestingly, the group was of mixed sex (although this may be related to the milder instability of these patients). Over 12 years of follow-up there was only one death which was not diabetes-related. The authors noted a tendency for DKA episodes to decline with the passage of time (and often retrospectively related to the alleviation of adverse psychosocial factors).

The London study[45] followed 13 patients, again with varying types of brittleness, over a relatively short duration (3–6 years). Five patients had severe recurrent DKA, and one died during follow-up, interestingly of profound hypoglycaemia at home. The authors noted that 'two other patients narrowly escaped death' – one also from hypoglycaemia, and one from severe DKA. Even with the relatively short follow-up period, a tendency for spontaneous improvement was again noted.

The Newcastle report[46] was of 20 young women with pure recurrent DKA, followed for a mean 8.2 years. There were 2 deaths (10%) – one from DKA, and one (possibly arrhythmic) during an operation to implant an intraperitoneal infusion cannula. Of the survivors, 10

(50%) were considered no longer brittle, and a further 4 had improved. For the whole group, mean (± SEM) insulin daily dose had significantly reduced (145 ± 46 units/day to 69 ± 18 units/day, p <0.005), as had annual hospital admissions (14.5 ± 10.5 to 1.9 ± 2.9, p <0.001). The authors noted that resolution of brittleness 'at least in some cases seemed to coincide with positive life events such as marriage, pregnancy, or forming a stable relationship.'

The longest duration and largest outcome study was, however, that of Kent et al.[3] In this report, a total of 33 young females with recurrent DKA were identified from original assessments in the late 1970s and early to mid 1980s at the Freeman Hospital, Newcastle-upon-Tyne, and Guy's Hospital, London. Information on 26 patients was available 10 years later. As well as examining mortality figures and causes, the patients and their hospitals were visited by a diabetes research nurse for structured quantitative and qualitative assessment. Their clinical, life quality and complication status was also compared in a case-control way, with a group of stable type 1 patients, matched for age, sex and diabetes duration.

Of the 26 patients, 5 had died (19%) – only one from DKA (and largely due to lack of venous access). Two died outside hospital – one from probable hypoglycaemia, the other possibly from a hyperkalaemic cardiac arrest due to chronic renal failure. The other 2 died suddenly in hospital: one probably hypoglycaemic, and the other perioperatively. The survivors, however, showed marked improvement, with brittleness resolving in 90% at 10 years. For the whole group of survivors there were significant falls in daily insulin dose, hospitalizations and DKA episodes. Positive life events again often coincided with improvement. For example, the authors recorded one consultant's comments: 'She seems to have settled into an uneventful life following her marriage; she has not been admitted for some years now and at one stage was in every fortnight.'

As well as the significant mortality risk, resolution occurred at the expense of a considerable diabetic complication burden. At initial assessment no patients had complications, but at 10-year follow-up, 14 of the 21 survivors (67%) were affected – 13 with retinopathy (1

Table 3.3 Pregnancy outcome in 21 females with recurrent DKA followed for 10 years (combined London and Newcastle series). Data are means ± SD[3]

	Recurrent DKA patients	Stable type 1 controls
Number	21	20
Age (years)	29 ± 6	32 ± 5
Duration diabetes (years)	18 ± 5	17 ± 4
Total pregnancies	28	27
Live healthy infants	15 (54%)	25 (95%)
Miscarriages	10 (48%)	2 (10%)
Stillbirths	1 (5%)	0 (0%)
Malformation	2 (1%)*	0 (0%)

* Both malformations were serious, and one (a complex cardiac defect) was fatal.

registered blind), 6 with neuropathy, 2 with nephropathy and 2 with cataracts. Of particular concern and significance was the adverse pregnancy outcomes which occurred in this group – they are compared with the stable control group of type 1 diabetic patients in Table 3.3.

The strong message from all these studies is that recurrent DKA tends to resolve spontaneously in time with life improvement. However, there is a significant mortality risk, and complications cost.

Managing recurrent DKA

Managing a condition with so complex an aetiology is clearly difficult, and a 'cure' is rarely a viable option. Treatment difficulties are

Table 3.4 Management options for patients with severe recurrent DKA

1. **Survival options**
   Continuous intravenous insulin infusion (CIVII)[52]
   Continuous intraperitoneal insulin infusion (CIPII)[53,54]
   Implantable insulin infusion pumps (IP or IV)[55]
   Pancreatic transplantation[56]

2. **Curative possibilities**
   Removal from causative stress (if present)[7,48]
   Psychoanalytical approaches[49]
   Cognitive analytical therapy (CAT)[50,51]

3. **Expectant approaches**
   'Masterly inactivity'[43]

(Adapted from reference 28.)

compounded at presentation to tertiary referral centres, as patients are usually significantly overweight and overinsulinized, and may be habituated (or even 'addicted') to non-compliant behaviour. Treatment of metabolic decompensation at this stage is frequently also severely hampered by lack of peripheral (and sometimes even central) venous access.

Treatment options are outlined in Table 3.4. The assessment and management coordinator should be an expert diabetologist, preferably with previous experience of patients with recurrent DKA. True organic causes of recurrent DKA are extraordinarily rare, but nevertheless occult infection and endocrinopathies (e.g. thyrotoxicosis) should be quickly excluded. A diabetes specialist nurse should review in detail the patient's self-treatment techniques and educational understanding of diabetes. A home visit (even if the patient is in hospital) and family assessment are often useful at this stage. As mentioned previously, unless there is a specific reason, psychiatric assessment is unlikely to be helpful; but the involvement of a clinical psychologist can be useful.[21] Intensive interviews and enquiries by the coordinating diabetologist are, however, of paramount importance – past experience suggests that it is the lead clinician who most commonly uncovers factitious behaviour.[21,22,47]

When serious manipulation with treatment is found, it should be openly discussed with the patient (although not in a judgemental and confrontational manner). It must be realized, however, that such discussions rarely, if ever, in themselves lead to a magical return to more compliant behaviour. If recurrent DKA is being self-induced to escape from an intolerable stress, then clearly removal from that situation may be helpful. Thus, in one of the earliest descriptions of the syndrome, Peck and Peck in 1956[7] reported a case due to intolerable family abuse, where removal from the family (the patient went to live with an aunt) led to a dramatic and immediate return to good glycaemic control on lower insulin doses, with no episodes of DKA. Unfortunately, scenarios such as this are relatively uncommon, although, more recently, removal to residential care in similar cases has been reported to be of use.[48] When there are no such recognizable psychosocial precipitants, psychoanalytical techniques should be explored. They have proved useful in some cases,[49] and there is a particular evidence base for the use of cognitive analytical therapy (CAT) in recurrent DKA[50,51] (for further details see Chapter 11). These treatment options do however require expert psychologists with an interest and experience of unstable and poorly compliant diabetic patients.

Given that the majority of patients with recurrent DKA resolve spontaneously with time, a policy of 'masterly inactivity'[43] (see Table 3.4) may be a viable option. The difficulty is, however (as discussed in the previous section), that there is also a significant mortality and morbidity risk with time.[3] Venous access difficulties can also make episodes of DKA especially dangerous, and life-preserving 'mechanistic' options may have to be considered (see Table 3.4). In the past these have involved continuous intravenous insulin infusion (CIVII)

57

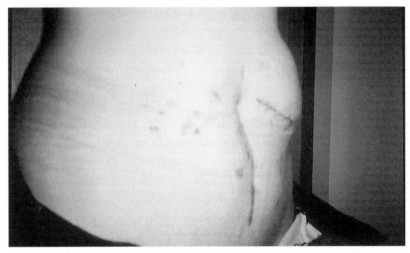

Figure 3.3 *Refractory, life-threatening brittle diabetes with recurrent DKA. The patient had no accessible peripheral veins, as well as bilaterally thrombosed subclavian veins and left femoral vein. The abdomen shows multiple scars from intraperitoneal lines attached to external insulin pumps, a previous failed internal pump implantation, and a current 'Infusaid' pump implanted on the left side of the abdomen. Remarkably the patient survived, and is now well on subcutaneous insulin.*

or continuous intraperitoneal insulin infusion (CIPII) by external pump.[52,53] The difficulty with such techniques as these is their tendency to complications. Both can cause local sepsis, and the external components of the systems are prone to patient interference. CIVII can be associated with septicaemia and subclavian vein thrombosis, and CIPII with peritonitis and line blockage by fibrinous plugs (although recent experience does show more favourable outcomes than earlier reports[54]). Perhaps more attractive options currently are continuous intravenous or intraperitoneal infusion from a fully implantantable insulin pump,[55] segmental pancreatic transplantation[56] or perhaps islet transplantation. All these methods are 'closed' and therefore protected from patient interference, and infection is less of a problem. Nevertheless, they are 'brave treatments' which should not be undertaken lightly, although on occasions they have alleviated critically life-threatening situations[57](Figure 3.3). These options are fully discussed in Chapter 13.

Conclusions

Young female type 1 diabetic patients with the syndrome of recurrent DKA represent one of the greatest therapeutic challenges in clinical diabetology. Although clearly a small minority of type 1 patients, they probably represent the extreme end of a syndrome of maladaptation and poor compliance. Thus, interesting recent studies from Dundee in Scotland have compared the prescription and consumption of insulin in a large number of young type 1 diabetic patients.[58] A significant discrepancy was found in 28%, with the amount of insulin used being considerably less than the doses prescribed. These patients had poorer glycaemic control and more admissions with DKA. Other studies have shown that insulin omission is common in young women in general with type 1 diabetes,[59] and especially in those with eating disorders.[60]

Interestingly, a new cause of insulin omission and DKA has emerged in the last few years – that of intravenous drug abuse and type 1 diabetes. The literature is scant, but one study has shown more frequent episodes of DKA in intravenous drug users (IVDU),[61] usually related to insulin omission while 'high' on intravenous drugs. Another report has confirmed this finding, and also demonstrated an excess of microvascular complications and infection-related admissions.[62]

The cause of repeated DKA attacks in IVDU patients is of course understandable, but the more typical young female patients with recurrent DKA remain aetiologically and therapeutically problematic. No literature exists on preventive aspects of this syndrome and indeed there are probably few if any clinical opportunities. However, at-risk young women with type 1 diabetes can be potentially identified, and in these patients there should be a high index of suspicion for adverse psychosocial factors, possible eating disorders and treatment non-compliance. Overinsulinization should be avoided at all costs. Despite this, patients with recurrent DKA will from time to time appear, and will challenge the skill, patience and dedication of the diabetes care team.

References

1. Gill GV. The spectrum of brittle diabetes. J Roy Soc Med 1992; 85: 259–61.
2. Gill GV, Lucas S, Kent LA. Prevalence and characteristics of brittle diabetes in Britain. Quart J Med 1996; 89: 839–43.
3. Kent LA, Gill GV, Williams G. Mortality and outcome of patients with brittle diabetes and recurrent ketoacidosis. Lancet 1994; 344: 778–81.
4. Hinkle LE, Wolf S. Experimental study of life situations, emotions and the occurrence of acidosis in a juvenile diabetic. Am J Med 1949; 217: 130–5.
5. Rosen H, Lidz T. Emotional factors in the precipitation of recurrent diabetic acidosis. Psychosom Med 1949; 11: 211–15.
6. Hinkle LE, Wolf S. Importance of life stress in course of management of diabetes mellitus. JAMA 1952; 148: 513–20.
7. Peck FB, Peck FB. Tautologous diabetic coma – a behaviour syndrome. Multiple unnecessary episodes of diabetic coma. Diabetes 1956; 5: 44–7.
8. Tattersall R. Brittle diabetes. Clin Endocrinol Metab 1977; 6: 403–19.
9. Gale E, Tattersall R. Brittle diabetes. Br J Hosp Med 1979; 21: 589–97.
10. Gill GV, Husband DJ, Walford S et al. Clinical features of brittle diabetes. In: Pickup JC, ed, Brittle diabetes. Blackwell, Oxford, 1985, pp 29–40.
11. Gill GV, Walford S, Alberti KGMM. Brittle diabetes – present concepts. Diabetologia 1985; 228: 579–89.
12. Pickup J, Williams G, Johns P, Keen H. Clinical features of brittle diabetic patients unresponsive to optimised subcutaneous insulin therapy (continuous subcutaneous insulin infusion). Diabetes Care 1983; 6: 279–84.
13. Flexner CW, Weiner JP, Saudek CD, Dans PE. Repeated hospitalisation for diabetic ketoacidosis. The game of "Sartoris". Am J Med 1984; 76: 691–5.
14. Fulop M. Recurrent diabetic ketoacidosis. Am J Med 1985; 78: 54–60.
15. Schade DS, Drumm DA, Duckworth WC, Eaton RP. The etiology of incapacitating brittle diabetes. Diabetes Care 1985; 8: 12–20.
16. Schade DS, Eaton P, Drumm DA, Duckworth WC. A clinical algorithm to determine the etiology of brittle diabetes. Diabetes Care 1985; 8: 5–11.
17. Dandona P, Foster M, Healey F, Greenbury E, Beckett AG. Low dose insulin infusions in patients with high insulin requirements. Lancet 1978; 2: 283–5.
18. Pickup JC, Howe PD, Bilous RW, Alberti KGMM, Keen H. Management of severely brittle diabetes by continuous subcutaneous and intramuscular infusion: evidence for a defect in subcutaneous insulin absorption. Br Med J 1981; 282: 347–50.
19. Friedenberg GR, White N, Cataland S et al. Diabetes responsive to intravenous but not subcutaneous insulin: effectiveness of aprotinin. N Engl J Med 1981; 305: 363–8.

UNIVERSITY OF WOLVERHAMPTON
Walsall Learning Centre

ITEMS ISSUED:

Customer ID: 7605348919

Title: ABC of diabetes
ID: X6214784962
Due: 11/03/2009 23:59

Title: renal system
ID: 7624339694X
Due: 11/03/2009 23:59

Title: Unstable and brittle diabetes
ID: 7624295641R
Due: 25/03/2009 23:59

Total items: 3
04/03/2009 16:16
Total Items on Loan: 3
Overdue: 0

Thank you for using Self Service
Please keep your receipt

Overdue books are fined at 40p per day for
1 week loans, 10p per day for long loans.

UNIVERSITY OF WOLVERHAMPTON
Walsall Learning Centre

ITEMS ISSUED:

Customer ID: 7605348919

Title: ABC of diabetes
ID: 7621478465
Due: 11/03/2009 23:59

Title: renal system
ID: 762433894X
Due: 11/03/2009 23:59

Title: Unstable and brittle diabetes
ID: 7624299618
Due: 25/03/2009 23:59

Total items: 3
04/03/2009 16:16
Total Items on Loan: 3
Overdue: 0

Thank you for using Self Service.
Please keep your receipt.

Overdue books are fined at 40p per day for
1 week loans, 10p per day for long loans.

20. Williams G, Pickup JC, Clark AJL et al. Changes in blood flow close to subcutaneous insulin injection sites in stable and brittle diabetes. Diabetes 1983; 32: 466–73.
21. Gill GV, Walford S, Alberti KGMM. Brittle diabetes – all in the mind? Diabetologia 1984; 27: 279A.
22. Schade DS, Duckworth WC. In search of the subcutaneous insulin resistance syndrome. N Engl J Med 1986; 315: 147–53.
23. Massi-Benedetti M, Home PD, Gill GV et al. Hormonal and metabolic responses in brittle diabetic patients during feedback intravenous insulin infusion. Diabet Res Clin Pract 1987; 3: 307–13.
24. Williams G, Pickup JC, Keen H. Massive insulin resistance apparently due to rapid decrease of circulating insulin. Am J Med 1987; 82: 1247–52.
25. Husband DJ, Pernet A, Gill GV, Hanning I, Alberti KGMM. The metabolic response to insulin deprivation in idiopathic brittle diabetes. Diabet Res 1986; 3: 193–8.
26. Taylor R, Husband DJ, Marshall SM, Tunbridge WMG, Alberti KGMM. Adipocyte insulin binding and insulin sensitivity in "brittle" diabetes. Diabetologia 1984; 27: 441–6.
27. Taylor R, Hetherington CS, Gill GV, Alberti KGMM. Changes in tissue insulin sensitivity in previously "brittle" diabetes. Hormon Metab Res 1986; 18: 493.
28. Gill GV. Does brittle diabetes exist? In: Gill GV, Pickup JC, Williams G, eds, Difficult diabetes. Blackwell Science, Oxford, 2000, pp 151–67.
29. Schade DS. Brittle diabetes: strategies, diagnosis and treatment. Diabet Metab Rev 1998; 4: 371–90.
30. Drumm DA, Schade DS. How communication disorders destabilise diabetes. Clin Diabet 1986; 4: 16.
31. Crystal D. Profiling linguistic disability. Edward Arnold, London, 1982.
32. Kemmar FW, Bisping R, Steingruber HJ et al. Psychological stress and metabolic control in patients with type 1 diabetes mellitus. N Engl J Med 1986; 314: 1078–84
33. Pernet A, Walker M, Gill GV, Orskov H, Alberti KGMM. Metabolic effects of adrenaline and noradrenaline in man: studies with somatostatin. Diabet Metab 1984; 10: 98–105.
34. Steel JM. Such a nice girl. Lancet 1994; 344: 365–6.
35. Faulkner W. Sartoris. Harcourt Brace, New York, 1929.
36. Favazza AR, Conterio K. Female habitual self-mutilators. Acta Psychiatr Scand 1989; 79: 283–9.
37. Steel JM, Young RJ, Lloyd GG, Clarke BF. Clinically apparent eating disorders in young diabetic women associated with painful neuropathy and other complications. Br Med J 1987; 284: 859–62.
38. Joseph B. Addiction to near death. Int J Psycho-Analysis 1982; 63: 449–56.
39. Naish JM. Problems of deception in medical practice. Lancet 1979; 2: 139–42.

40. Ayres JG, Miles JF, Barnes PJ. Brittle asthma. Thorax 1998; 53: 315–21.
41. Gill GV, Williams G. Brittle Addison's disease: a new variation on a familiar theme. Postgrad Med J 2000; 76: 166–7.
42. Gill GV, Walford S. The fragile female diabetic. Diabet Med 1986; 3: 284.
43. Gill GV, Williams G. Brittle diabetes. In: Alberti KGMM, Zimmet P, De Fronzo RA, eds. International Textbook of Diabetes Mellitus, 2nd edn. John Wiley, Oxford, 1997, pp 1123–33.
44. Tattersall R, Gregory R, Selby C, Kerr D, Heller S. Course of brittle diabetes: 12 year follow-up. Br Med J 1991; 302: 1240–3.
45. Williams G, Pickup JC. The natural history of brittle diabetes. Diabet Res 1988; 7: 13–18.
46. Gill GV, Alberti KGMM. Outcome of brittle diabetes. Br Med J 1991; 303: 285–6.
47. Schade DS, Drumm DD, Eaton RP, Sterling WA. Factitious brittle diabetes mellitus. Am J Med 1985; 78: 777–84.
48. Geffken GR, Lewis C, Johnson SB et al. Residential care for youngsters with difficult-to-manage insulin dependent diabetes. J Paed Endocrinol Metab 1997; 10: 517–27.
49. Fonogy P, Moran GS. A psychoanalytical approach to the treatment of brittle diabetes in children and adolescents. In: Hodes M, Mooney S, eds, Psychological treatment in disease and illness. Gaskell and the Society for Psychosomatic Research, London, 1993, pp 166–92.
50. Ryle A, Boa C, Fosbury J. Identifying the causes of poor self-management in insulin-dependent diabetes: the use of cognitive analytic therapy techniques. In: Hodes M, Mooney S, eds, Psychological treatment in disease and illness. Gaskell and the Society for Psychosomatic Research, London, 1993, pp 157–65.
51. Fosbury JA, Bosley CM, Ryle A, Sonksen PH, Lowy C. Cognitive analytic therapy with poorly controlled type 1 diabetic patients. Diabetologia 1994; 37 (suppl 1): A175.
52. Bayliss J. Brittle diabetes: long-term control with a portable, continuous intravenous insulin infusion system. Br Med J 1981; 283: 1207–9.
53. Pozza G, Spotti D, Micossi P et al. Long-term continuous intra-peritoneal insulin treatment in brittle diabetes. Br Med J 1983; 286: 255–6.
54. DeVries JH, Eskes SA, Snoek FJ et al. Continuous intraperitoneal insulin infusion in patients with "brittle" diabetes: favourable effects on glycaemic control and hospital stay. Diabet Med 2002; 19: 496–501.
55. Gill GV, Husband DJ, Wright PD et al. The management of severe brittle diabetes with "Infusaid" implantable pumps. Diabet Res 1986; 3: 135–7.
56. Du Toit DF, Heydenrych JJ, Coetzee AR, Weight M. Pancreatic transplantation in a patient with severe insulin resistance. S Afr Med J 1988; 73: 723–5.
57. Gill GV, Kent L, Williams G, Walford S, Alberti KGMM. An unusual case of relapsing brittle diabetes. Pract Diabet 1995; 12: 38–9.

58. Morris AD, Boyle DIR, McMahon AD et al. Adherence to insulin treatment, glycaemic control, and ketoacidosis in insulin-dependent diabetes mellitus. Lancet 1997; 350: 1505–10.

59. Polonsky WH, Aponte JE, Anderson BJ et al. Insulin omission in women with IDDM. Diabetes Care 1994; 17: 1178–85.

60. Jones JM, Lawson ML, Daneman D, Olmsted MP, Rodin G. Eating disorders in adolescent females with and without type 1 diabetes: cross sectional study. Br Med J 2000; 320: 1563–6.

61. Warner EA, Greene GS, Buchsbaum MS, Cooper DS, Robinson BE. Diabetic ketoacidosis associated with cocaine use. Arch Int Med 1998; 158: 1799–802

62. Saunders SA, Martin J, Democratis J, MacFarlane IA. Intravenous drug abuse in type 1 diabetes: massive financial and healthcare implications. Diabet Med 2003; 20 (suppl 2): 101.

chapter 4

Insulin resistance in diabetes

Balasubramanian Ravikumar and Roy Taylor

Introduction

Resistance to insulin was first described more than 60 years ago, when some patients with diabetes were noted to be less sensitive to insulin treatment than others.[1] The development of the radioimmunoassay (RIA) technique for the measurement of insulin by Berson and Yalow started the modern study of insulin resistance in man. Insulin resistance describes an impaired biological response to insulin.[2] It has been broadly defined as 'a state (of a cell, tissue, or organism) in which a greater than normal amount of insulin is required to elicit a quantitatively normal response'.[3,4] However, insulin resistance can be selective – i.e. involving only certain aspects of insulin action – a fact that complicates both the definition and its characterization in vivo and in vitro.[5] This chapter will focus on the clinical effects of insulin resistance on type 1 diabetes, its role in obesity and type 2 diabetes, and possible ways of modifying insulin resistance. The underlying pathophysiology of insulin resistance and in-vivo assessment of insulin sensitivity will also be discussed.

Clinical implications of insulin resistance

Insulin resistance in type 1 diabetes and adolescence

Although insulin resistance is invariably associated with type 2 diabetes, it plays a role in type 1 diabetes. It is important to recognize that insulin resistance is merely a convenient term to refer to the state of relatively low insulin sensitivity. There is a wide range of insulin sensitivity in health[6] and this variation is clinically important in type 1 diabetes. For instance, it determines the daily insulin dose requirements. Athletes in training tend to require low dosage because of high insulin sensitivity related to physical fitness. Likewise, weight loss improves insulin sensitivity and lower insulin doses are required. If Addison's disease develops, insulin sensitivity rises as cortisol levels fall and hypoglycaemia becomes frequent unless insulin doses are sharply decreased. In contrast, insulin sensitivity decreases during intercurrent illness, the postoperative period, and during steroid administration. This is reflected in increasing insulin dose requirements. For instance, high-dose steroid therapy requires an immediate increase in insulin dose by about 40%.[7] If this is not done then gross hyperglycaemia supervenes.

Clinical presentation and natural course of type 1 diabetes

Differences in insulin action at different times during the natural course of type 1 diabetes may partly explain the different clinical characteristics observed, especially during adolescence and in unstable brittle diabetic patients. In the prediabetic period, the degree of insulin sensitivity may affect rates of progression to frank hyperglycaemia. The usual onset of type 1 diabetes in adolescence and during illnesses, when insulin sensitivity is decreased, further supports this notion. In a prospective study of 15 newly diagnosed type 1 diabetic patients, Yki-Jarvinen et al[8] showed that insulin action was markedly impaired at 2 weeks after diagnosis. However, 3 months later, insulin sensitivity was no longer different to that of controls. This period coincided with the often-observed clinical remission or 'honeymoon phase'. It was also seen that insulin sensitivity was inversely related to the glycated haemoglobin (HbA_{1c}) level, implying that antecedent hyperglycaemia may decrease insulin action (glucose toxicity). Chronic hyperglycaemia or 'glucose toxicity' causes insulin resistance by stimulation of the hexosamine pathway of glucose metabolism, with consequent desensitization of the glucose transport mechanism.[9] The initial improvement in insulin sensitivity seen in the early course of type 1 diabetes is short-lived. Subsequently, the sensitivity to insulin deteriorates, so that by 10 or more years of diabetes it is about 60% of normal.[8] The observation that the loss of remission period is related to decreased insulin sensitivity further exemplifies the importance of insulin sensitivity in the natural course of the illness.[10]

Insulin resistance in adolescent type 1 diabetes

Impaired insulin action in adolescent type 1 patients is an important contributor to poor glycaemic control in these subjects. A number of

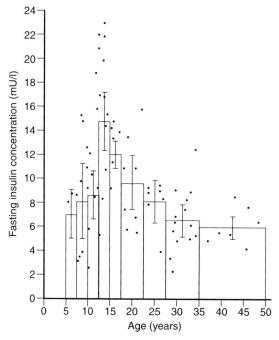

Figure 4.1 *Insulin sensitivity during puberty. Fasting plasma insulin concentrations increase during puberty, only returning to prepubertal levels in early adulthood. The bars indicate the mean values with 95% confidence intervals for different age groups.*[12]

67

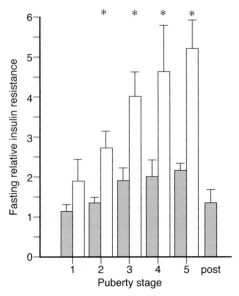

Figure 4.2 *Fasting relative insulin resistance in adolescent diabetes. Comparison of fasting insulin resistance in diabetic patients (no shading) relative to normal adolescents (dark shading) at the end of a glucose clamp study. During puberty, the diabetic patients are more insulin resistant than the normal adolescents at every stage; *p<0.02.[14]*

studies have shown a decrease in insulin sensitivity in normal puberty[11,12] (Fig. 4.1) and this is thought to be due to alterations in insulin action in peripheral tissues.[13] This normal pubertal decrease in insulin sensitivity is accentuated in type 1 diabetic patients[14] (Fig. 4.2). The change in insulin sensitivity in puberty is thought to be secondary to puberty-associated growth hormone (GH) secretion. In a group of children and young adults with type 1 diabetes, Acerini et al showed that insulin sensitivity varied with age, the lowest being in adolescence, and was inversely related to overnight GH concentrations.[15] The insulin antagonistic effect of GH is thought to be principally mediated through defective peripheral glucose metabolism. Thus, treatment of type 1 diabetes during puberty is a therapeutic challenge for physiological as well as behavioural reasons. Despite using measures such as increasing insulin doses and intensive multiple-dose regimens, the overall impact on glycaemic control, as judged by HbA_{1c}, has been generally disappointing.[16,17] In addition, intensive regimens pose problems during puberty because of the increased risk of nocturnal hypoglycaemia and weight gain.

Over-insulinization

Occasionally, continuation of the higher insulin doses from adolescence into early adulthood life leads to the over-insulinization syndrome. This is characterized by unpredictable swings between hyperglycaemia and hypoglycaemia in individuals who are taking insulin doses in excess of 1.5 units/kg. A single-step decrease of insulin dose by approximately 50% and close liaison with a diabetes specialist nurse abolishes the swings. It may be hypothesized that insulin itself is altering insulin receptor function. Follow-up of such individuals confirms that insulin dose requirements do not return to levels required during adolescence. The over-insulinization syndrome is a clinical diagnosis to be suspected in young adults taking high insulin doses and exhibiting swinging blood glucose control. Clearly, the differential diagnosis of poor compliance must also be considered in such circumstances, although the subsequent clinical course is very different in such cases.

Brittle diabetes

Changes in insulin sensitivity can cause unpredictable swings in blood glucose control in some patients. In a group of 6 young women labelled as having 'brittle' diabetes, Taylor et al showed that adipocytes displayed resistance to insulin stimulation as a consequence of reduced adipocyte insulin receptor affinity, but without any changes in insulin receptor number.[18] However, following 3–6 months of stable control using intraperitoneal and insulin pump therapy, the decreased adipocyte insulin sensitivity and adipocyte insulin receptor affinity were reversed.[19] Hence, the observed changes in tissue insulin sensitivity seen in these subjects must have been secondary to metabolic derangements caused by markedly fluctuating and high insulin doses given during the preceding period of poor control.

Pathophysiology of insulin resistance in type 1 diabetes

The pathophysiology of insulin resistance in type 1 diabetes is poorly understood. Postprandial suppression of hepatic glucose output is grossly defective in type 1 diabetes.[20] Moreover, the liver of patients with poorly controlled type 1 diabetes fails to take up glucose and store it as glycogen, as has been demonstrated by magnetic resonance spectroscopy[21] (Fig. 4.3). This increases delivery of glucose to peripheral tissues, where the capacity of muscle (and adipose tissue) to remove glucose is also severely compromised secondary to impaired insulin action. This multifactorial defective insulin action in type 1 diabetes leads to a marked defect in glucose disposal, with consequent hyperglycaemia and renal glycosuria. In states of relative insulin deficiency, hyperglycaemia, glycosuria and volume depletion stimulate the secretion of a variety of counter-regulatory hormones

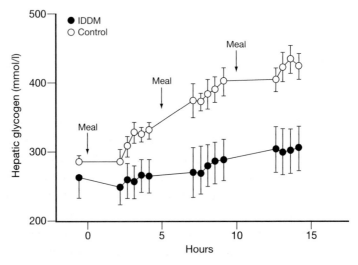

Figure 4.3 *Defective net hepatic glycogen synthesis in type 1 diabetes. Time course for hepatic glycogen concentration (mmol/l) in both normal and type 1 diabetic subjects during the course of a day in which three isocaloric mixed meals were ingested 5 hours apart. By 15 hours the type 1 diabetic subjects synthesized only 30% of the glycogen that was synthesized by the control group (p<0.05).[21]*

(glucagon, catecholamines, growth hormone and cortisol), which further augment hepatic gluconeogenesis and ketogenesis.[22] Decreased insulin sensitivity, compounded by counter-regulatory hormone excess and with relative insulin deficiency, conspires to precipitate diabetic ketoacidosis.

Obesity, type 2 diabetes and insulin resistance

The association of obesity with type 2 diabetes has been recognized for decades, and the major factor linking these together is the ability of obesity to engender insulin resistance. Large epidemiological studies have revealed that the risk of diabetes rises as body fat content (as assessed by body mass index) increases from the very lean to the very obese.[23] The effect of enlarged adipose tissue mass in decreasing insulin sensitivity is an area of expanding research and several mediators have been implicated in bridging this link.

Insulin resistance in the natural history of type 2 diabetes

The relative contributions of impaired insulin sensitivity and impaired insulin secretion to the aetiology of type 2 diabetes is a subject of intense debate. The majority of patients with type 2 diabetes are obese and insulin resistant. Insulin resistance in obesity and type 2 diabetes is manifest by decreased insulin-stimulated glucose transport and metabolism in adipocytes and skeletal muscle and by impaired suppression of hepatic glucose output.[24] Reduced insulin sensitivity and defective cellular mechanisms of skeletal muscle insulin sensitivity (see below) have been confirmed in type 2 diabetes and in normoglycaemic offsprings of type 2 diabetes. Thus, the presence of these abnormalities in these normal individuals suggests that insulin resistance is a primary factor in the development of type 2 diabetes. In the presence of obesity and a family history of type 2 diabetes, insulin resistance is typically present and increased insulin secretion, especially after meals, compensates for the reduced insulin sensitivity. However, when β-cell function declines, hyperglycaemia ensues as the compensatory mechanism fails. Thus, a distinct prediabetic phase exists, comprising of compensatory β-cell function and insulin resistance. It is at this stage of the disease process where current prevention studies are hoping to delay the onset of type 2 diabetes.[25,26]

Adipose tissue depots and insulin resistance

The significance of the location of body fat to insulin resistance has lately been of prime focus. Central (intra-abdominal) depots of fat are much more strongly linked with insulin resistance, type 2 diabetes and cardiovascular disease than are peripheral (i.e. subcutaneous) fat depots.[27] The exact cause for this intriguing difference is unclear, although the direct delivery of fatty acids from visceral fat to the liver, higher lipolytic activity of abdominal adipocytes with consequent difference in free fatty acid fluxes and the differences in secretion of adipokines between fat depots are all possible mechanisms.

The cellular mechanisms and genetics of type 2 diabetes are considered later in this chapter. From a clinical standpoint, weight loss and improvement of insulin sensitivity remain the major therapeutic targets for the treatment of type 2 diabetes. The demonstration of improved insulin sensitivity by exercise and weight reduction is unequivocal.[28,29] Diabetes prevention strategies, as seen in the Finnish Diabetes Prevention Study, illustrate the role of lifestyle modifications in modulating the pathogenesis of diabetes.[25]

Insulin resistance and the metabolic syndrome

Over the years hyperglycaemia has been linked to a number of metabolic abnormalities. As early as 1923, Kylin[30] observed the link between hyperglycaemia, hypertension and gout. Reaven[31] reintroduced this concept of clustering of metabolic abnormalities with insulin resistance, leading to increased cardiovascular risk in humans, and termed it 'syndrome X'. In 1998, the World Health Organization (WHO) proposed a unifying definition of this syndrome and chose to call it the 'metabolic syndrome'.[32] The number of components of this syndrome have steadily grown (Table 4.1). The links between obesity and insulin resistance have been discussed in the preceding section and the other associations will be briefly discussed.

Table 4.1 Metabolic and cardiovascular risk factors associated with the metabolic syndrome

Insulin resistance

Obesity

Dyslipidaemia: high triglyceride levels, low HDL cholesterol levels, increased small and dense LDL cholesterol particles and increased Apo B levels

Hypertension

Microalbuminuria

Abnormalities in coagulation: increased fibrinogen levels and increased plasminogen activator inhibitor-1 (PAI) levels

Endothelial dysfunction and accelerated atherosclerosis

Insulin resistance and dyslipidaemia

The association between insulin resistance and abnormal lipoprotein metabolism may partly help explain the increased cardiovascular risk with insulin-resistant states.[33,34] The characteristic features of the dyslipidaemia associated with insulin resistance include hypertriglyceridaemia, low HDL (high-density lipoprotein) cholesterol and increased small dense LDL (low-density lipoprotein) particles. In addition to hypertriglyceridaemia, there is increased postprandial triglyceride concentrations and postprandial accumulation of highly atherogenic remnant lipoproteins,[35] thereby conferring an increased risk of atherogenesis and cardiovascular risk.

Insulin resistance and hypertension

Although a weaker association than dyslipidaemia, hypertension is associated with insulin resistance and adds significantly to the overall risk of cardiovascular disease. Approximately 50% of insulin-resistant individuals are hypertensive. The possible mechanisms may include overactivity of the sympathetic nervous system,[36] activation of the renin–angiotensin system, increased reabsorption of sodium and water by the kidney,[37] and possibly defective vasodilatation relating to impaired insulin action on the vasculature.

Insulin resistance and microalbuminuria

Microalbuminuria is a common feature of the metabolic syndrome and is a strong predictor of cardiovascular mortality. Recent evidence suggests that microalbuminuria may even be a predictor for the onset of type 2 diabetes.[38] In the Botnia study, amongst the various risk factors for cardiovascular mortality in the metabolic syndrome, microalbuminuria conferred the strongest risk of cardiovascular death.[39]

Insulin resistance and abnormalities of coagulation

Prothrombotic and fibrinolytic factors act in concert to maintain haemostasis. The levels of plasminogen activator inhibitor-1, a prothrombotic factor, has been found to be high in insulin resistance, and highly correlated with an increased risk of myocardial infarction.[40] In addition, the insulin-resistant state is also characterized by hyper-fibrinogenaemia, a further prothrombotic state.

Insulin resistance and endothelial dysfunction and accelerated atherosclerosis

The degree of insulin sensitivity is directly related to carotid artery intimal thickness[41] and hence atherosclerosis. Adherence of circulating monocytes to the endothelium herald the formation of lipid-laden foam cells, the precursor of the atherosclerotic plaque. In a group of healthy volunteers without diabetes, the binding of monocytes to the endothelium was highly correlated to the degree of insulin sensitivity,[42] thus suggesting an important role for insulin in endothelial function and prevention of atherosclerosis.

Modifying insulin resistance

As insulin resistance is a modifiable feature of type 2 diabetes, the relative effectiveness of possible treatments is important to consider.

Currently no pharmacological agents are licensed to treat insulin resistance in the absence of diabetes. From a clinical standpoint, a number of non-pharmacological measures improve insulin sensitivity: namely, calorie-restricted diet, weight reduction and exercise. This section will deal with the pharmacological treatment of insulin resistance in type 2 diabetes.

Metformin

Despite extensive research, the precise cellular mechanism of metformin action is still not clearly understood. The possible mechanisms of action of metformin include predominantly suppression of endogenous glucose output[43,44] and modest changes in peripheral insulin sensitivity.[45]

Elevated basal endogenous glucose production (EGP) and non-suppression of EGP following meal ingestion contribute to fasting and postprandial hyperglycaemia, respectively, in type 2 diabetes. Most studies have shown metformin to inhibit EGP,[43,46] in the presence of unaltered or reduced plasma insulin concentrations.[47] This is predominantly due to decreased gluconeogenesis,[44] although decreased glycogenolysis is also likely to contribute.[48] Recently, Inzucchi and colleagues, using meal tolerance tests and hyperinsulinaemic–euglycaemic clamp studies with tracer infusion, demonstrated that following 3-month monotherapy with metformin the predominant effect of metformin was on EGP, and improvement in peripheral insulin sensitivity was small[49] (Fig. 4.4). The improvement in glucose disposal with metformin was also comparable with what was observed in sulphonylurea treatment alone.[50,51] This suggests that the small effect on peripheral glucose disposal by metformin is more likely to be a consequence of improved insulin sensitivity secondary to improved blood glucose levels[52] rather than a direct effect of metformin.

The interpretation of the mode of action of metformin is confounded by the improvement in glycaemic control and reduction of body weight, which can both influence insulin sensitivity. In addition, a modest anorectic effect has been postulated to contribute to its efficacy. Other cellular mechanisms, such as decreased free fatty

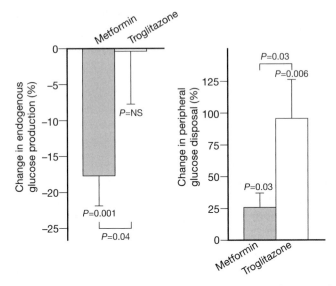

Figure 4.4 *Mechanism of action of metformin and troglitazone. Changes in hepatic glucose production and insulin stimulated glucose disposal rate in subjects with type 2 diabetes under hyperinsulinaemic-clamp conditions following 3-month monotherapy with metformin or troglitazone (cross-over design). Data are given as percentage change from pretreatment levels.*[49]

acids (FFAs) release from adipose tissue and reduced lipid oxidation, have not been supported by recent studies.[44,53]

The use of metformin in insulin-resistant states without diabetes has been of interest recently. Several studies have demonstrated that treatment with metformin has a favourable effect in women with polycystic ovary syndrome (PCOS), where insulin resistance plays an important role. In a recent review on insulin sensitivity and fertility, data from 6 studies examining the effect of metformin treatment in PCOS were reviewed, and a 15–50% decrease in plasma insulin and serum testosterone levels was observed in these studies.[54] There has also been recent debate on the use of metformin to prevent or delay the onset of diabetes. The recent Diabetes Prevention Programme study, comparing the prevention of diabetes with metformin against lifestyle interventions, showed that lifestyle intervention, and, to a lesser extent, metformin, were both successful in preventing diabetes.[26] However, the routine use of metformin in non-diabetic obese or impaired glucose tolerance (IGT) subjects is not currently recommended.

Thiazolidinediones

Thiazolinediones (TZDs) or glitazones are a new class of oral hypogly-caemic agents that improve glycaemia through improved insulin sensi-tivity. TZDs are synthetic ligands of the nuclear hormone receptor peroxisome proliferator activated receptor-γ (PPAR-γ), which is predominantly expressed in adipocytes, intestine and macrophages.[55] PPARs are a family of nuclear receptors comprising three subtypes (α, γ and δ). They are ligand-dependent transcription factors that regulate target gene expression by binding to specific response elements present in regulatory regions of the target genes. The endogenous ligands for this receptor are currently unknown. The therapeutic effects of TZDs clearly suggest that PPAR-γ regulates insulin sensitivity in diabetes. The effect of TZDs on improving insulin sensitivity, primar-ily peripheral insulin sensitivity[49] (Fig. 4.4), has been cited to be the cause of their effect on glycaemic control, and hence they are referred to as 'insulin sensitizers'. The site of action and molecular targets of PPAR-γ are unclear. Both adipose tissue[56] and skeletal muscle[57] have been suggested as potential target sites, although the evidence for a primary effect on triglyceride metabolism is strong.[58] Recent evidence suggests that the improvement in insulin sensitivity may be secondary to redistribution of fat from visceral to subcutaneous adipose depots[59] and, hence, altered triglyceride metabolism.

Troglitazone, the first TZD, was withdrawn secondary to hepato-toxicity, although the two other available agents – rosiglitazone and pioglitazone – appear not to share this property and both are useful in improving glycaemic control in type 2 diabetes. Using the hyper-insulinaemic clamp technique, troglitazone[49] and pioglitazone[60] have been shown to improve peripheral insulin sensitivity. In addition to improving glucose metabolism, the TZDs also improve lipid metabo-lism and vascular endothelial function. The glitazones differ in their effects on lipid metabolism, the reasons for which are unknown. Pioglitazone has been shown to reduce triglyceride levels by about 9% and increase HDL cholesterol levels by 12–19%.[58] Rosiglitazone, however, had no lowering of triglycerides, although a rise in HDL levels have been observed.

Weight gain, dilutional anaemia and oedema are the common side effects. Reversible elevations of liver enzymes (alanine aminotransferase; ALT) may occur, although no serious hepatotoxicity has yet been reported with rosiglitazone or pioglitazone. In view of the weight gain and oedema, caution should be exercised in patients with congestive cardiac failure.

In summary, both rosiglitazone and pioglitazone have the potential not only to improve glycaemia but also to improve other components of the insulin resistance syndrome, including dyslipidaemia and hypertension, and thereby prevent or delay premature atherosclerotic cardiovascular disease. However, long-term studies are needed to determine whether these agents fulfil this potential.

Pathophysiology and pathogenesis of insulin resistance

Multiple sites of insulin resistance: muscle, liver and adipose tissue

Skeletal muscle

Insulin normally increases the uptake, storage and oxidation of glucose in skeletal muscle. The rate of insulin-stimulated glucose disposal is significantly slowed in insulin-resistant subjects.

Muscle glycogen metabolism. In healthy humans, after an overnight fast, approximately 1600 mmol of glycogen is stored in muscle,[61] compared with about 420 mmol in liver. Postprandial muscle glycogen storage measurements using ^{13}C-magnetic resonance spectroscopy (MRS),[62] revealed that 26–35% of ingested carbohydrate was stored in

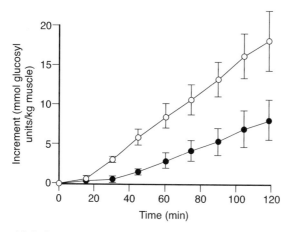

Figure 4.5 *Defective muscle glycogen synthesis in type 2 diabetes. Comparison of increments from baseline in muscle glycogen concentration in normal (open circles) and type 2 diabetic subjects (solid circles) during hyperglycaemic–hyperinsulinaemic clamp study. Values are means ± SE expressed per kilogram of muscle tissue.[63]*

muscle as muscle glycogen. In addition, muscle glycogen concentrations do not start to rise until 1–2 hours after eating, thus suggesting that the fate of glucose during this immediate postprandial period is oxidation, followed by glycogen synthesis. Recently, studies under hyperglycaemic–hyperinsulinaemic conditions showed that defective muscle glycogen synthesis played a major role in insulin resistance in type 2 diabetes[63] (Fig. 4.5). Further evidence of defective muscle glucose metabolism was shown using ^{13}C-MRS following a standard meal at breakfast and lunch. Despite considerably higher plasma insulin and glucose levels, muscle glycogen in diabetic individuals rose subnormally 4 hours following breakfast, when compared to controls (9% vs 31%), explaining a major portion of postprandial hyperglycaemia.[64]

Defects in glycogen synthase,[65–68] hexokinase[69,70] and glucose transport[71,72] have all been implicated in the subnormal muscle glycogen synthesis in type 2 diabetes. Recently, the relative importance of these steps to insulin-stimulated muscle glucose metabolism have been assessed by performing ^{13}C/^{31}P-MRS studies to measure intracellular concentrations of glucose, glucose-6-phosphate and glycogen in muscle of patients with type 2 diabetes and age–weight matched control subjects.[71] Intracellular glucose-6-phosphate is an intermediary metabolite between glucose transport and glycogen synthesis, and hence the relative activities of these two steps will be reflected by its intracellular concentration. In the event of decreased activity of glycogen synthase in diabetes, glucose-6-phosphate in diabetic patients would be expected to be increased relative to that of normal individuals. Using ^{31}P-MRS to assess intracellular glucose-6-phosphate under conditions of hyperglycemic–hyperinsulinaemia, an increase of approximately 0.1 mmol/l intracellular glucose-6-phosphate was observed in normal individuals but no change in patients with type 2 diabetes. The blunted incremental change of glucose-6-phosphate concentration in the type 2 diabetic patients in response to insulin stimulation can therefore be ascribed to either decreased glucose transport activity or decreased hexokinase II activity. Similar results were seen in insulin-resistant offspring of parents with type 2 diabetes.[73,74] Thus, even prior to the onset of diabetes, insulin-resistant offspring of patients with type 2 diabetes have decreased rates of muscle glycogen synthesis that are secondary to a defect in muscle glucose transport or hexokinase activity.

A novel ^{13}C-MRS method has recently been applied to assess intracellular glucose concentrations, a transient intermediary metabolite between glucose transport and glucose phosphorylation, to determine whether glucose transport or hexokinase II activity is the rate-controlling step for insulin-stimulated muscle glycogen synthesis in patients with type 2 diabetes.[75] If hexokinase II activity was decreased in diabetes relative to glucose transport activity, a substantial increase in intracellular glucose would be observed, whereas if glucose transport was primarily responsible for maintaining intracellular glucose metabolism, intracellular glucose and glucose-6-phosphate should change proportionately. It was observed that intracellular glucose concentration was far lower in the diabetic subjects than the value expected if hexokinase II was the primary rate-controlling enzyme for glycogen synthesis. These data indicate the major role of glucose transport in determining muscle glycogen synthesis in diabetes and its principal role in the pathogenesis of insulin resistance.

Decreased delivery of substrate or insulin to the tissue bed has been hypothesized to be at least partially responsible for the insulin resistance in type 2 diabetes.[76] No difference has been observed in the ^{13}C-MRS measured ratio of extra- to intracellular water space in normal subjects and diabetic patients, implying that insulin-mediated vasodilatation could not be responsible.

Overall, these results are consistent with the hypothesis that glucose transport is the rate-controlling step for insulin-stimulated muscle glycogen synthesis, and represents the major cause of insulin resistance in patients with type 2 diabetes. Hence, one can infer that agents that enhance hexokinase II or glycogen synthase activity will not be as effective in alleviating insulin resistance as any agent which primarily improves glucose transport.

Free fatty acids and skeletal muscle insulin resistance.   Insulin-resistant states (e.g. obesity and type 2 diabetes) are characterized by increased plasma FFAs.[77,78] Randle et al[79,80] originally proposed that the insulin resistance in obesity was a result of an increase in fatty acid oxidation. Recently, under euglycaemic–hyperinsulinaemic conditions, artificial elevation of plasma FFA concentrations in healthy subjects caused a reduction of 50% in insulin-stimulated rates of muscle glycogen synthesis, as observed by ^{13}C- and ^{31}P-MRS and a similar reduction of 50% in glucose oxidation.[74] The drop in muscle glycogen synthesis was preceded by a fall in intramuscular glucose-6-phosphate. This suggests that the increase in FFAs induces insulin resistance by inhibiting glucose transport and phosphorylation. Similar results have been obtained in obesity[81] and type 2 diabetes.[73] Dresner et al[82] used ^{13}C-MRS to evaluate intracellular glucose concentrations (as described earlier) in response to elevated FFAs and observed that this caused a significant reduction in intracellular glucose concentration, implying that the rate-controlling step for fatty acid-induced insulin resistance in humans is glucose transport. In addition, elevation of FFAs abolished the insulin-stimulated phosphatidylinositol

3-kinase (PI 3-kinase) activity, suggesting that defects in this signalling step or other preceding steps may account for the defective glucose transport by affecting the glucose transporter GLUT4 translocation.

In healthy non-diabetic women, the intramuscular triglyceride content determined by muscle biopsy was shown to be inversely related to insulin sensitivity.[83] This was also observed by Perseghin et al[84] in a cross-sectional study of young, normal-weight offspring of type 2 diabetes patients, in whom fasting plasma FFA concentration also displayed an inverse relationship to insulin sensitivity. More recently, measurements of intramuscular triglyceride content by muscle biopsy and ^{1}H-MRS showed a strong relationship between accumulation of intramyocellular triglyceride and insulin resistance. Hence, accumulation of intramuscular fatty acids or fatty acid metabolites appears to play an important role in determining sensitivity of insulin.

Liver

Insulin stimulates hepatic glucose uptake and suppresses endogenous glucose production (EGP) following a glucose load. Defective suppression of EGP in response to normal and elevated insulin levels suggests that insulin resistance may operate at the level of liver. However, the response of the liver to changes in the hormonal milieu depends on the mode of glucose delivery, and a response to an oral glucose load differs from that of a mixed meal or to that of an unphysiological condition of constant hyperinsulinaemia. A recent study in type 2 diabetic subjects[85] showed that in response to a mixed meal EGP was initially rapidly suppressed (0–60 min), but incomplete suppression of EGP contributed to the subsequent hyperglycaemia 60–240 minutes after the meal (Fig. 4.6). These observations were made under the normal day-to-day circumstances of elevated plasma glucose and glucagon, and suggest that insulin sensitivity of the liver in type 2 diabetes in the immediate postprandial state is normal. However, the ultimate degree of suppression of EGP is subnormal. It is known that the suppression of hepatic glucose production can be mediated by both direct and indirect effects of insulin.[86,87] Increased fatty acid supply is also known to increase EGP. It may be that the

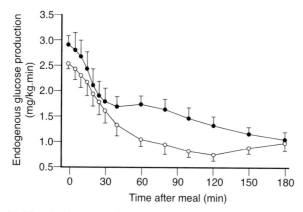

Figure 4.6 *Hepatic glucose production in type 2 diabetes following a mixed meal. Change in hepatic glucose production during the early post-meal phase in type 2 diabetes (solid circles) and matched normal subjects (open circles). Initial rapid suppression is followed by incomplete suppression of hepatic glucose production after 45 minutes.*[85]

increased fatty acid supply to the liver in diabetic patients increases the background level of gluconeogenesis, which is not immediately suppressible by insulin.

Overall, hepatic insulin resistance differs distinctly from that of muscle. In contrast to muscle, insulin resistance is less pronounced in the liver. This is not surprising, since glucose transport is the most insulin-insensitive step in skeletal muscle, whereas glucose transport is not rate limiting for hepatic glucose metabolism.

Adipose tissue

In addition to muscle and liver, adipose tissue is an important site of insulin action. Muscle has long been considered the major site of insulin-stimulated glucose uptake in vivo, with adipose tissue contributing 10-fold less to total body glucose disposal. Moreover, muscle mass is considerably greater than adipose tissue in non-obese humans. However, regulation of lipolysis – because of the release of glycerol and FFAs into the circulation – makes adipose tissue an important player in glucose homeostasis. As suggested above, FFAs and their metabolites play a crucial role in the pathogenesis of muscle insulin resistance. Both obesity and lipoatrophy cause insulin resistance and a predisposition to type 2 diabetes, demonstrating that adipose tissue is crucial in regulating metabolism beyond its ability to take up glucose. Severe insulin resistance observed in the transgenic models of lipodystrophic diabetes is remarkably reversed not only by fat transplantation into fatless mice[88] but also by infusion of leptin[89] and adiponectin.[90] These observations illustrate the important role of adipose tissue in influencing insulin sensitivity.

Cellular mechanisms of insulin resistance

The insulin resistance of obesity and type 2 diabetes is associated with defects at many levels of the insulin signalling pathway. The understanding of the cellular mechanisms has largely depended on targeted deletion of components of the insulin signalling pathway in vivo using homologous recombinations and more recently combinatorial knockouts which try to mimic polygenic type 2 diabetes with heterozygous deletions. The insulin signalling cascade can be briefly summarized as follows: insulin binds to a specific receptor on cellular surfaces, which stimulates autophosphorylation of the intracellular region of the receptor β subunit.[91] This stimulates the tyrosine kinase activity of the receptor and hence catalyses the phosphorylation of cellular substrate proteins such as members of the insulin receptor substrate (IRS) family. Upon tyrosine phosphorylation, these proteins interact with other signalling molecules, resulting in a diverse series of signalling pathways, including activation of PI-3 kinase and downstream phosphatidylinositol-3-phosphates-dependent kinases. The mitogen-activated protein (MAP) kinase cascade is then involved in protein synthesis and enzyme activation and deactivation, and gene expression, which act in a coordinated fashion to regulate vesicle trafficking and glucose transporter translocation.[92] The cellular mechanisms can be considered at each one of the following signalling steps.

Genetic defects in insulin receptor

Although rare, these conditions represent the most severe forms of insulin resistance, and are exemplified by leprechaunism, the

Rabson–Mendenhall syndrome and the type A syndrome of insulin resistance[93] (see below).

Immunological blockade of insulin receptor
Specific antibodies to the insulin receptor can block the active site and this is referred to as 'type B insulin resistance'. This is a rare condition, and has been described in association with systemic lupus erythematosus (SLE),[94] Hodgkin's disease and ataxia telangiectasia).[4,5,95]

Insulin receptor substrates (IRS) mutations
Specific IRS-1 and IRS-2 knockout mice have provided interesting observations. Whereas IRS-1 knockout mice were insulin-resistant but not hyperglycaemic, probably in part due to compensation by IRS-2,[96] IRS-2 knockout mice were severely hyperglycaemic due to abnormalities of peripheral insulin action and failure of β-cell secretion.[97] This phenotype has several similarities to type 2 diabetes in man and outlines the role of IRS proteins in the development of cellular insulin resistance and β-cell function.

PI-3 kinases and protein kinase B (PKB)
Decreased expression and phosphorylation levels of early signalling elements, namely PI-3 kinase and PKB, have been variably demonstrated in type 2 diabetic patients.[98,99] Future research and studies on other downstream regulators will aid the understanding of the metabolic effects on these signalling cascades and their role in type 2 diabetes.

Genetics of insulin resistance
Twin studies of type 2 diabetes, familial clustering of type 2 diabetes and the high prevalence of this disease in some ethnic groups have driven the quest for potential candidate genes for insulin resistance.

Insulin receptor mutations
Fatal, but fortunately rare syndromes such as leprechaunism and the Rabson–Mendelhall syndrome are characterized by the mutations of

both insulin receptor alleles.[93] Other insulin receptor mutations affecting only one insulin receptor allele are compatible with life and cause severe insulin resistance syndromes – called 'type A insulin resistance'. It is important to note that hyperglycaemia may not develop during young adulthood, even in the face of this severe insulin resistance. However, screening for insulin receptor mutations in type 2 diabetes is less rewarding, with about 1–5% of patients showing several insulin receptor mutations.[100,101]

Insulin receptor substrates mutations

IRS-1 and IRS-2 mutations have been described in humans with some impaired insulin action, but these are found in the same frequency in non-diabetic compared to diabetic individuals, hence ruling out a major role is development of type 2 diabetes.[102]

PI 3-kinase mutations

Studies of PI 3-kinase mutations have revealed mixed results. The Scandinavian insulin-resistant population had a frequency of approximately 30% heterozygous and 2% homozygous form of PI 3-kinase mutation,[103] but this mutation was absent in Japanese type 2 diabetes patients.[104] A major role for these mutations is therefore unlikely.

Other candidate genes

Mutations of GLUT4, glycogen synthase and liver glucokinase promoter (among others) have been identified, but these mutations are not associated with insulin resistance or type 2 diabetes, apart from in a very few cases. A large number of genes remain to be screened, and the current evidence shows that a large number of heterozygous mutations in insulin signalling molecules are present in a high frequency in human subjects, but are insufficient to cause insulin resistance or type 2 diabetes. This suggests a polygenic pathogenesis of the condition.

Genome scans

New diabetes-associated loci on different chromosomes have been identified on genome scans and these are mostly located in the vicinity of the known genes such as hepatic nuclear factor 1α (HNF 1α), the sulphonylurea receptor and the apolipoprotein A-2. These loci tend to be specific in certain ethnic groups, and they are probably less important in the common type 2 diabetic and insulin-resistant patients.

Assessing insulin sensitivity in vivo

Model assessments of insulin sensitivity

Minimal model assessment of insulin sensitivity

Minimal model assessment involves using individual patient data from frequently sampled intravenous glucose tolerance tests (FSIVGTT). Glucose causes insulin to rise, and insulin causes glucose to fall. The complex feedback can be analysed mathematically to calculate insulin sensitivity and β-cell function. The minimal model approach, introduced by Bergman et al,[105] computes estimates of insulin resistance and β-cell function for each profile, using curve-fitting techniques. In addition to insulin sensitivity, the minimal model yields a measure of the rate of glucose uptake stimulated by increased circulating glucose, independent of insulin action (a process called 'glucose effectiveness').

As endogenous insulin secretion is essential for calculations, modifications using intravenous tolbutamide[106] to augment second-phase insulin secretion and bolus injections of insulin[107] have been used successfully to assess insulin sensitivity in various groups of subjects. The advantages are that the FSIVGTT is less labour intensive than the clamp methodology (see below), and is a simple method for the assessment of insulin sensitivity. The estimates from the minimal model approach correlate well with those from the euglycaemic clamp methodology (see below).[108]

Homeostatic model assessment (HOMA)

It is possible to derive an indication of insulin sensitivity from fasting plasma glucose and fasting plasma insulin/C peptide levels. Matthews et al[109] derived a mathematical model (HOMA) that takes into account the effect of hyperglycaemia on plasma insulin levels. The results obtained are qualitatively different from other indices, as it related mainly to the feedback effect of insulin in controlling fasting hepatic glucose output (basal insulin sensitivity). Provided that the analysis of both plasma insulin and glucose levels are undertaken with scrupulous care, the index obtained correlates well with estimates from the euglycaemic clamp.[110] The method is simple and is appropriate for assessing insulin sensitivity in groups of patients over long periods of time.

Euglycaemic–hyperinsulinaemic clamp

The euglycaemic–hyperinsulinaemic clamp technique has become regarded as the gold standard against which other methods are validated.[111] Insulin is infused intravenously at a steady rate and arterial plasma glucose is measured every 5 minutes. Glucose is infused intravenously at a rate that maintains a constant plasma glucose concentration. If insulin sensitivity is high, as in an athlete, a high rate of glucose infusion will be needed. If insulin sensitivity is low, as in a patient with type 2 diabetes, then only low rates of glucose infusion will be needed. The average glucose infusion rate over at least 30 minutes after an apparent steady state is reached (usually 2 hours) is taken as the index of insulin sensitivity.

Insulin clamps give relatively assumption-free estimates of insulin resistance, with a high degree of reproducibility (although in the absence of appropriate tracer techniques, it assumes that the EGP is shut off by insulin infusion). In addition, it is possible to combine other measurements such as indirect calorimetry or to perform tissue biopsies at known plasma insulin levels.[112] Measurements of arteriovenous differences across a limb or volume of other tissue allows measurements in local tissues. In addition, MRS can be combined with clamps to track both flux and the change in absolute levels of glycogen stores and intermediary compounds.[63]

The limitations are that the clamp, in its simplest version, offers a point estimate of insulin action with one substrate (glucose), and one stimulus (insulin concentration at steady state). To maintain the necessary steady state of plasma glucose a high degree of skill is required. Full dose–response curves for in-vivo insulin-mediated glucose uptake have been constructed by multiple euglycaemic[113] or hyperglycaemic clamps[114] sequentially or on different days, but this approach is labour intensive and is not suitable for larger groups of subjects. Clamps reflect insulin sensitivity during high plasma insulin levels and not necessarily that of the fasting state, when hepatic glucose production and non-insulin-dependent tissues exert major influences on glucose homeostasis. Moreover, the clamps typically use insulin at levels above those that normal individuals experience and may therefore fail to reveal potential abnormalities of processes regulated by lower insulin concentrations. Conceptually, it is assumed that measurements are made at a steady state, but in reality only the plasma glucose and, perhaps, the glucose infusion rates are steady. Inside the major metabolic organs, the process of substrate storage steadily progresses, and the situation is clearly unphysiological. Nevertheless, some epidemiological studies have successfully utilized the clamp method, such as in Pima Indians[115] and in the European Group for Study of Insulin Resistance (EGIR) study. This method has also been the fundamental basis of assessment of insulin action in target tissues – such as muscle, adipose tissue and the liver. It has also found its place in attempts to identify 'insulin resistance genes'.

Insulin infusion sensitivity tests: short insulin tolerance test (ITT)

This simple test provides an assessment of insulin sensitivity and is becoming widely used as a rapid and reliable measure. It can be combined with other measures such as indirect calorimetry. Insulin at a dose of 0.1–0.15 mU/kg is injected as an intravenous bolus. Arterial plasma glucose is used as the index of insulin sensitivity. The results agree well with those from clamp studies ($r = 0.81$–0.86),[116] and reflect the sensitivity of both liver and muscle to insulin-induced suppression of hepatic glucose output and stimulation of glucose uptake. This is the ideal test if a measure of insulin sensitivity only is required. It is also ideal for studying large populations, as it is simple and is least dependent on operator skill.

Conclusion

Our understanding of the complex pathogenesis and genetics of diabetes has been greatly influenced by the concept of insulin resistance. The natural history of both type 1 and type 2 diabetes is critically dependent upon changes in insulin sensitivity. Changes in insulin sensitivity determine the clinical features of type 1 diabetes and influence the dose changes required during the course of the disease. As evident from the recent diabetes prevention studies, it is clear that changes in insulin sensitivity can have a significant impact on delaying the onset of type 2 diabetes. A clear understanding of insulin resistance is therefore vital to formulating rational treatment modalities for treating diabetes at all stages. As the quest for novel agents to improve insulin sensitivity gathers momentum, it is possible that the complex pathogenesis of type 2 diabetes may soon be unravelled.

References

1. Himsworth H. Diabetes mellitus: a differential into insulin-sensitive and insulin-insensitive types. Lancet 1936; 1: 127–30.
2. Yalow RS, Berson SA. Plasma insulin concentrations in nondiabetic and early diabetic subjects: determinations by a new sensitive immunoassay technique. Diabetes 1960; 9: 254–60.
3. Hunter SJ, Garvey T. Insulin action and insulin resistance: diseases involving defects in insulin receptors, signal transduction and glucose transport effector system. Am J Med 1998; 5: 331–46.
4. Mantzoros CS, Flier JS. Insulin resistance: the clinical spectrum. In: Mazzaferi E, ed., Advances in endocrinology and metabolism, Vol. 6. Mosby-Year Book, St Louis, 1995.
5. Moller DE, Flier JS. Insulin resistance: mechanisms, syndromes, and implications. N Engl J Med 1991; 325: 938–48.
6. Lillioja S, Mott DM, Howard BV et al. Impaired glucose tolerance as a disorder of insulin action: longitudinal and cross sectional studies in Pima Indians. N Engl J Med 1988; 318: 1217–25.

7. Dashora U, Taylor R. In: DJ Betteridge, ed., Fifty cases of diabetes. Martin Dunitz, London, 2002; 17–20.
8. Yki-Jarvinen H, Koivisto VA. Natural course of insulin resistance in type I diabetes. N Engl J Med 1986; 315: 224–30.
9. Marshall S, Garvey T, Traxinger RR. New insights into the metabolic regulation of insulin action and insulin resistance: role of glucose and amino acids. FASEB J 1991; 5: 3031–6.
10. Hramiak IM, Dupre J, Finegood DT. Determinants of clinical remission in recent-onset IDDM. Diabetes Care 1993; 16: 125–32.
11. Amiel SA, Sherwin RS, Simonson DC, Lauritano AA, Tamborlane WV. Impaired insulin action in puberty. A contributing factor to poor glycaemic control in adolescents with diabetes. N Engl J Med 1986; 315: 215–19.
12. Smith CP, Dunger DB, Williams AJK et al. Relationship between insulin, insulin-like growth factor-I and dehydroepiandosterone sulphate concentrations during childhood, puberty and adult life. J Clin Endocrinol Metab 1989; 68: 932–7.
13. Amiel SA, Caprio S, Sherwin RS et al. Insulin resistance of puberty: a defect restricted to peripheral glucose metabolism. J Clin Endocrinol Metab 1991; 72: 277–82.
14. Dunger DB, Edge JA. Diabetes and puberty. In: Marshall SM, Home PD, eds., The diabetes annual, Vol. 10. Elsevier Science, Amsterdam, 1996.
15. Acerini CL, Cheetham TD, Cheetham JA, Edge JA, Dunger DB. Both insulin sensitivity and insulin clearance in children and young adults with type 1 (insulin-dependent) diabetes vary with growth hormone concentrations and with age. Diabetologia 2000; 43: 61–8.
16. Mann NP, Johnston DI. Total glycated haemoglobin (HBA1c) levels in diabetic children. Arch Dis Child 1982; 57: 434–7.
17. Smith C, Dunger DB, Mitten S et al. A comparison of morning and bed-time ultralente administration when using multiple injections in adolescence. Diabet Med 1988; 5: 352–5.
18. Taylor R, Husband DJ, Marshall SM, Tunbridge WMG, Alberti KGMM. Adipocyte insulin binding and insulin sensitivity in brittle diabetes. Diabetologia 1984; 27: 441–6.
19. Taylor R, Hetherington CS, Gill GV, Alberti KGMM. Changes in tissue insulin sensitivity in previously brittle diabetics. Horm Metabol Res 1986; 18: 493.
20. Wahren J, Felig P, Cerasi E, Luft R. Splanchnic and peripheral glucose and amino acid metabolism in diabetes mellitus. J Clin Invest 1972; 51: 1870–8.
21. Hwang J-H, Perseghin G, Rothman DL et al. Impaired net hepatic glycogen synthesis in insulin-dependent diabetic subjects during mixed meal ingestion. J Clin Invest 1995; 95: 783–7.
22. Shamoon H, Hendler R, Sherwin RS. Altered responsiveness to cortisol,

epinephrine, and glucagon in insulin-infused juvenile-onset diabetics. A mechanism for diabetic instability. Diabetes 1980; 29: 284–91.

23. Colditz GA, Willett WC, Stampfer MJ et al. Weight as a risk factor for clinical diabetes in women. Am J Epidemiol 1990; 132: 501–13.

24. Reaven GM. Pathophysiology of insulin resistance in human disease. Physiol Rev 1995; 75: 473–86.

25. Uusitupa M, Louheranta A, Lindstrom J et al. The Finnish Diabetes Prevention Study. Br J Nutr 2000; 83 (suppl 1): S137–42.

26. Knowler WC, Barrett-Connor E, Fowler SE et al. Diabetes Prevention Program Research Group. Reduction in the incidence of type 2 diabetes with lifestyle intervention or metformin. N Engl J Med 2002; 346: 393–403.

27. Kissebah AH, Krakower GR. Regional adiposity and morbidity. Physiol Rev 1994; 74: 761–811.

28. Kelley DE. Effects of weight loss on glucose homeostasis in NIDDM. Diabet Rev 1995; 3: 366–77.

29. Schneider SH, Morgado A. Effects of fitness and physical training on carbohydrate metabolism and associated risk factors in patients with diabetes. Diabet Rev 1995; 3: 378–407.

30. Kylin E. Studien ueber das Hypertonie-Hyperglykaemie-Hyper-urikamesyndrom. Zentralblatt fuer Innere Medizin 1923; 44: 105–27.

31. Reaven GM. Role of insulin resistance in human disease. Diabetes 1988; 37: 1595–607.

32. Alberti KGMM, Zimmet PZ for the WHO Consultation. Definition, diagnosis and classification of diabetes mellitus, provisional report of a WHO consultation. Diabet Med 1998; 15: 539–53.

33. Fontbonne A, Eschwege E, Cambien F et al. Hypertriglyceridemia as a risk factor of coronary heart disease mortality in subjects with impaired glucose tolerance or diabetes. Diabetologia 1989; 32: 300–4.

34. Grundy SM. Hypertriglyceridemia, insulin resistance, and the metabolic syndrome. Am J Cardiol 1999; 83: 25–9F.

35. Kim H-S, Abbasi F, Lamendola C, McLaughlin T, Reaven GM. Effect of insulin resistance on postprandial elevations of remnant lipoprotein concentrations in postmenopausal women. Am J Clin Nutr 2001; 74: 592–5.

36. Landsberg L. Insulin resistance and hypertension. Clin Exp Hypertens 1999; 21: 885–94.

37. DeFronzo RA, Cooke CR, Andres R, Faloona GR, Davis PJ. The effect of insulin on renal handling of sodium, potassium, calcium, and phosphate in man. J Clin Invest 1975; 55: 845–55.

38. Mykkanen L, Haffner SM, Kuusisto J, Pyorala K, Laakso M. Microalbu-minuria precedes the development of NIDDM. Diabetes 1994; 43: 552–7.

39. Isomaa B, Almgren P, Tuomi T et al. Cardiovascular morbidity and mortality associated with the metabolic syndrome. Diabetes Care 2001; 24: 683–9.

40. Juhan-Vague I, Alessi MC, Vague P. Increased plasminogen activator inhibitor-1 levels: a possible link between insulin resistance and atherothrombosis. Diabetologia 1991; 34: 457–62.
41. Howard G, O'Leary DH, Zaccaro D et al. Insulin sensitivity and atherosclerosis: the Insulin Resistance Atherosclerosis Study Investigators. Circulation 1996; 93: 1809–17.
42. Chen N-G, Abassi F, Lamendola C et al. Mononuclear cell adherence to cultured endothelium is enhanced by hypertension and insulin resistance in healthy nondiabetic volunteers. Circulation 1999; 100: 940–3.
43. Johnson AB, Webster JM, Sum CF et al. The impact of metformin therapy on hepatic glucose production and skeletal muscle glycogen synthase activity in overweight Type II diabetic patients. Metabolism 1993; 42: 1217–22.
44. Stumvoll M, Nurjhan N, Perriello G, Dailey G, Gerich JE. Metabolic effects of metformin in non-insulin-dependent diabetes mellitus. N Engl J Med 1995; 333: 550–4.
45. Fery F, Plat L, Balasse EO. Effects of metformin on the pathways of glucose utilization after oral glucose in non-insulin-dependent diabetes mellitus patients. Metabolism 1997; 46: 227–33.
46. DeFronzo RA, Barzilai N, Simonson DC. Mechanism of metformin action in obese and lean non-insulin-dependent diabetes. J Clin Endocrinol Metab 1991; 73: 1294–301.
47. DeFronzo RA, Goodman AM. Efficacy of metformin in patients with non-insulin dependent diabetes mellitus. The Multicentre Metformin Study group. N Engl J Med 1995; 333: 541–9.
48. Cusi K, Consoli A, DeFronzo RA. Metabolic effects of metformin in non-insulin-dependent diabetes mellitus. J Clin Endocrinol Metab 1996; 81: 4059–67.
49. Inzucchi SE, Maggs DG, Spollett GR et al. Efficacy and metabolic effects of metformin and troglitazone in Type II diabetes mellitus. N Engl J Med 1998; 338: 867–72.
50. Sheu WH, Jeng CY, Fuh MM, Chen YD, Reaven GM. Effect of glipizide treatment on response to an infused glucose load in patients with NIDDM. Diabetes Care 1995; 18: 1582–7.
51. Vestergaard H, Weinreb JE, Rosen AS et al. Sulphonylurea therapy improves glucose disposal without changing skeletal muscle GLUT4 levels in non insulin dependent diabetes mellitus subjects: a longitudinal study. J Clin Endocrinol Metab 1995; 80: 270–5.
52. Rossetti L, Smith D, Shulman GI, Papachristou D, Defronzo RA. Correction of hyperglycaemia with phlorizin normalizes tissue sensitivity to insulin in diabetic rats. J Clin Invest 1987; 79: 1510–15.
53. Riccio A, Del Prato S, Vigili de Kreutzenberg S, Tiengo A. Glucose and lipid metabolism in non-insulin-dependent diabetes: effect of metformin. Diabet Metab 1991; 17: 180–4.

54. Taylor R, Marsden PJ. Insulin sensitivity and fertility. Human Fertility 2000; 3: 65–9.

55. Lemberger T, Braissant O, Juge AC et al. PPAR tissue distribution and interactions with other hormone-signaling pathways. Ann NY Acad Sci 1996; 804: 231–51.

56. Rieusset J, Auwerx J, Vidal H et al. Regulation of gene expression by activation of the peroxisome proliferator-activated receptor gamma with rosiglitazone (BRL-49653) in human adipocytes. Biochem Biophys Res Commun 1999; 265: 265–71.

57. Park KS, Ciaraldi TP, Carter LA et al. Troglitazone regulation of glucose metabolism in human skeletal muscle cultures from obese type 2 diabetic subjects. J Clin Endocrinol Metab 1998; 83: 1636–43.

58. Shaffer S, Rubin CJ, Zhu E. The effects of pioglitazone on the lipid profile in patients with type 2 diabetes [Abstract]. Diabetes 2000; 48(suppl): 508P.

59. Miyazaki Y, Mahankali A, Matsuda M et al. Effect of pioglitazone on abdominal fat distribution and insulin sensitivity in type 2 diabetic patients. J Clin Endocrinol Metab 2002; 87: 2784–91.

60. Kawamori R, Matsuhisa M, Kinoshita J et al. Pioglitazone enhances splanchnic glucose uptake as well as peripheral glucose uptake in non-insulin-dependent diabetes mellitus. AD-4833 Clamp-OGL Study Group. Diabet Res Clin Pract 1998; 41: 35–43.

61. Taylor R, Magnussen I, Rothman DL et al. Direct assessment of liver glycogen storage by ^{13}C-nuclear magnetic resonance spectroscopy and regulation of glucose homeostasis after a mixed meal in normal subjects. J Clin Invest 1996; 97: 126–32.

62. Taylor R, Price TB, Katz LD, Shulman RG, Shulman GI. Direct measurement of change in muscle glycogen concentration after a mixed meal in normal subjects. Am J Physiol 1993; 265: E224–9.

63. Shulman GI, Rothman DL, Jue T et al. Quantitation of muscle glycogen synthesis in normal subjects and subjects with non-insulin dependent diabetes by ^{13}C nuclear magnetic resonance spectroscopy. N Engl J Med 1990; 322: 223–8.

64. Carey PE, Halliday J, Snaar JE, Morris PG, Taylor R. Direct assessment of muscle glycogen storage after mixed meals in normal and type 2 diabetic subjects. Am J Physiol Endocrinol Metab 2003; 284(4): E688–94

65. Bogardus C, Lillioja S, Stone K, Mott D. Correlation between muscle glycogen synthase activity and in vivo insulin action in man. J Clin Invest 1984; 73: 1185–90.

66. Johnson AB, Argyraki M, Thow JC et al. Impaired activation of muscle glycogen synthase in non-insulin dependent diabetes mellitus is unrelated to the degree of obesity. Metabolism 1991; 40: 252–60.

67. Johnson AB, Argyraki M, Thow JC et al. The effect of sulphonylurea therapy on skeletal muscle glycogen synthase activity and insulin secre-

tion in newly presenting non-insulin dependent diabetic patients. Diabet Med 1991; 8: 243–53.

68. Wright KS, Beck-Nielsen H, Kolterman OG, Mandarino LJ. Decreased activation of skeletal muscle glycogen synthase by mixed meal ingestion in NIDDM. Diabetes 1988; 37: 436–40.

69. Braithewaite SS, Plazuk B, Colca JR, Edwards CW, Hofmann C. Reduced expression of hexokinase II in insulin-resistant diabetes. Diabetes 1995; 44: 43–8.

70. Kruszynska YT, Mulford MI, Baloga J, Yu JG, Olefsky JM. Regulation of skeletal muscle hexokinase II by insulin in nondiabetic and NIDDM subjects. Diabetes 1998; 47: 1107–13.

71. Rothman DL, Shulman RG, Shulman GI. ^{31}P Nuclear magnetic resonance measurements of muscle glucose-6-phosphate – evidence for reduced insulin dependent muscle glucose transport or phosphorylation activity in NIDDM. J Clin Invest 1992; 89: 1069–75.

72. Bonadonna RC, Del Prato S, Bonora E. Role of glucose transport and glucose phosphorylation in muscle insulin resistance of NIDDM. Diabetes 1996; 45: 915–25.

73. Rothman DL, Magnusson I, Cline G et al. Decreased muscle glucose transport/phosphorylation is an early defect in the pathogenesis of non-insulin-dependent diabetes mellitus. Proc Natl Acad Sci USA 1995; 92: 983–7.

74. Roden M, Price TB, Perseghin G et al. Mechanism of free fatty acid-induced insulin resistance in humans. J Clin Invest 1996; 97: 2859–65.

75. Cline GW, Petersen KF, Krssak M et al. Decreased glucose transport as a cause of decreased insulin-stimulated muscle glycogen synthesis in Type 2 diabetes. N Engl J Med 1999; 341: 240–6.

76. Yang YJ, Hope ID, Ader M, Bergman RN. Insulin transport across capillaries is rate limiting for insulin action in dogs. J Clin Invest 1989; 84: 1620–8.

77. Frayn K. Insulin resistance and lipid metabolism. Curr Opin Lipidol 1993; 4: 197–204.

78. Reaven GM, Hollenbeck C, Jeng C-Y, Wu MS, Chen YD. Measurement of plasma glucose, free fatty acid, lactate, and insulin for 24h in patients with NIDDM. Diabetes 1988; 37: 1020–4.

79. Randle PJ, Garland PB, Hales CN, Newsholme EA. The glucose fatty acid cycle: its role in insulin sensitivity and the metabolic disturbances of diabetes mellitus. Lancet 1963; i: 785–9.

80. Randle PJ, Kerbey AL, Espinal J. Mechanisms decreasing glucose oxidation in diabetes and starvation: role of lipid fuels and hormones. Diabet Metab Rev 1988; 4: 623–38.

81. Petersen KF, Hendler R, Price T et al. ^{13}C/^{31}P NMR studies on the mechanism of insulin resistance in obesity. Diabetes 1998; 47: 381–6.

82. Dresner A, Laurent D, Marcucci M et al. Effects of free fatty acids on

glucose transport and IRS-1-associated phosphatidylinositol 3-kinase activity. J Clin Invest 1999; 103: 253–9.

83. Phillips DIW, Caddy S, Ilic V et al. Intramuscular triglyceride and muscle insulin sensitivity: evidence for a relationship in nondiabetic subjects. Metabolism 1996; 45: 947–50.

84. Perseghin G, Scifo P, De Cobelli F et al. Intramyocellular triglyceride content is a determinant of in vivo insulin resistance in humans: a ^{1}H-^{13}C nuclear magnetic resonance spectroscopy assessment in offspring of type 2 diabetic parents. Diabetes 1999; 48: 1600–6.

85. Singhal P, Caumo A, Carey PE, Cobelli C, Taylor R. Regulation of endogenous glucose production after a mixed meal in type 2 diabetes. Am J Physiol 2002; 283(2): E275–83.

86. Lewis GF, Giacca A, Vranic M, Steiner G. Direct and indirect effects of insulin on hepatic glucose and very low density lipoprotein (VLDL) production. Curr Opin Endocrinol Diabet 1998; 5: 235–45.

87. Lewis GF, Zinman B, Groenewoud Y, Vranic M, Giacca A. Hepatic glucose production is regulated both by direct hepatic and extra hepatic effects of insulin in humans. Diabetes 1996; 45: 454–62.

88. Gavrilova O, Marcus-Samuels B, Graham D et al. Surgical implantation of adipose tissue reverses diabetes in lipoatrophic mice. J Clin Invest 2000; 105: 271–8.

89. Shimomura I, Hammer RE, Ikemoto S, Brown MS, Goldstein JL. Leptin reverses insulin resistance and diabetes mellitus in mice with congenital lipodystrophy. Nature 1999; 401: 73–6.

90. Yamauchi T, Kamon J, Waki H et al. The fat derived hormone adiponectin reverses insulin resistance associated with both lipoatrophy and obesity. Nature Med 2001; 7: 941–6.

91. Kauga M, Karlssson FA, Kahn CR. Insulin stimulates the phosphorylation of the 95,000-dalton subunit of its own receptor. Science 1982; 215: 185–7.

92. Saltiel AR, Kahn CR. Insulin signaling and regulation of glucose and lipid metabolism. Nature 2001; 414: 799–806.

93. Taylor SI, Arioglu E. Syndromes associated with insulin resistance and acanthosis nigricans. Basic Clin Physiol Pharmacol 1998; 9: 419–39.

94. Kellett HA, Collier A, Taylor R et al. Hyperandrogenism, insulin resistance, acanthosis nigricans, and systemic lupus erythematosus associated with insulin receptor antibodies. Metabolism 1988; 37: 656–9.

95. Baird JS, Johnson JL, Elliott-Mills D, Opas LM. Systemic lupus erythematosus with acanthosis nigricans, hyperpigmentation, and insulin receptor antibody. Lupus 1997; 6: 275–8.

96. Araki E, Lipes MA, Patti ME et al. Alternative pathway of insulin signaling in mice with targeted disruption of the IRS-1 gene. Nature 1994; 372: 186–90.

97. Withers DJ, Gutierrez JS, Towery H et al. Disruption of IRS-2 causes type 2 diabetes in mice. Nature 1998; 391: 900–4.

98. Krook A, Roth RA, Jiang XJ, Zierath JR, Wallberg-Henriksson H. Insulin stimulated Akt kinase activity is reduced in skeletal muscle from NIDDM subjects. Diabetes 1998; 47: 1281–6.

99. Bjornholm M, Kawano Y, Lehtihet M, Zierath JR. Insulin receptor substrate-1 phosphorylation and phosphatidylinositol 3-kinase activity in skeletal muscle from NIDDM subjects after in vivo insulin stimulation. Diabetes 1997; 46: 524–7.

100. O'Rahilly S, Choi WH, Patel P et al. Detection of mutations in insulin-receptor gene in NIDDM patients by analysis of single-stranded conformation polymorphisms. Diabetes 1991; 40: 777–82.

101. Kahn CR, Vicent D, Doria A. Genetics of non-insulin-dependent (type II) diabetes mellitus. Ann Rev Med 1996; 47: 509–31.

102. Almind K, Bjorbaek C, Vestergaard H et al. Amino acid polymorphisms of insulin receptor substrate-1 in non-insulin-dependent diabetes mellitus. Lancet 1993; 342: 828–32.

103. Hansen T, Anderson CB, Echwald SM et al. Identification of a common amino acid polymorphism in the p85 alpha regulatory subunit of phosphatidylinositol 3-kinase: effects on glucose disappearance constant, glucose effectiveness, and the insulin sensitivity index. Diabetes 1997; 46: 494–501.

104. Kawanishi M, Tamori Y, Masugi J et al. Prevalence of a polymorphism of the phosphatidylinositol 3-kinase p85 alpha regulatory subunit (codon 326 Meth→Ile) in Japanese NIDDM patients [Letter]. Diabetes Care 1997; 20: 1043.

105. Bergman RN, Ider YZ, Bowden CR, Cobelli C. Quantitative estimation of insulin sensitivity. Am J Physiol 1979; 236: E667–77.

106. Yang Y, Youn J, Bergman RN. Modified protocols improve insulin sensitivity estimation using the minimal model. Am J Physiol 1987; 253: E595–602.

107. Finegood DT, Hramiak IM, Dupre J. A modified protocol for estimation of insulin sensitivity with the minimal model of glucose kinetics in patients with insulin dependent diabetes. J Clin Endocrinol Metab 1990; 70: 1538–49.

108. Beard J, Bergman RN, Ward W, Porte DJ. The insulin sensitivity index in nondiabetic man: correlation between clamp-derived and IVGTT-derived values. Diabetes 1986; 35: 362–9.

109. Matthews DR, Hosker JP, Rudenski AS et al. Homeostasis model assessment: insulin resistance and β-cell function from fasting plasma glucose and insulin. Diabetologia 1985; 28: 412–19.

110. Bonora E, Targher G, Alberichie M et al. Homeostasis model assessment closely mirrors the glucose clamp technique in the assessment of insulin sensitivity: studies in subjects with various degrees of glucose tolerance and insulin sensitivity. Diabetes Care 2000; 23: 57–63.

111. DelPrato S, Ferrannini E, DeFronzo RA. Evaluation of insulin sensitivity

in man In: Clarke WL, Larner J, Pohl SL, eds., Methods in diabetes research: clinical methods, Vol. 2. John Wiley & Sons, New York, 1986.

112. Johnson AB, Argyraki M, Thow JC et al. Impaired activation of muscle glycogen synthase in non-insulin dependent diabetes mellitus is unrelated to the degree of obesity. Metabolism 1991; 40: 252–60.

113. Rizza RA, Mandarino LJ, Gerich JE. Dose–response characteristics for effects of insulin on production and utilization of glucose in man. Am J Physiol 1981; 240: E630–9.

114. DeFronzo RA, Ferrannini E. Influence of plasma glucose and insulin concentration on plasma glucose clearance in man. Diabetes 1982; 31: 683–8.

115. Lillioja S, Mott DM, Spraul M et al. Insulin resistance and insulin secretory dysfunction as precursors of non-insulin dependent diabetes mellitus. N Engl J Med 1993; 329: 1988–92.

116. Akinmokun A, Selby PL, Ramaiya K, Alberti KGMM. The short insulin tolerance test for determination of insulin sensitivity: a comparison with the euglycaemic clamp. Diabet Med 1992; 9: 432–7.

chapter 5

Subcutaneous insulin resistance, learning disabilities and unstable diabetes

Denise A Drumm and David S Schade

Introduction

Subcutaneous insulin resistance is a term coined to denote a pathogenic mechanism causing unstable diabetes.[1-15] The term implies that the affected diabetic patient is unable to absorb insulin normally because the subcutaneous tissue contains a substance or a characteristic that prevents the normal absorption of insulin. The logical result would be the inability to control diabetes when insulin is injected subcutaneously. Conversely, the term subcutaneous insulin resistance implies that the diabetes control should be good when the insulin is given by another route (usually intravenous). This chapter will focus on the following issues:

■ When does subcutaneous insulin resistance exist?
■ What are alternative explanations for the clinical reports of subcutaneous insulin resistance?

- How does manipulative behaviour differ from factitious disease in unstable diabetes?
- What are learning disabilities and why do they cause unstable diabetes?
- What is the current status of subcutaneous insulin resistance as a pathogenic mechanism for unstable diabetes?

When does subcutaneous insulin resistance exist?

The subcutaneous tissue is arguably the worst location into which to deliver insulin into the human body. There are several reasons supporting this statement. First, the subcutaneous tissue is not a uniform structure. It is composed of many types of tissues, including adipocytes, melanocytes, fibrocytes, blood vessels (large and small), hair follicles, circulating red and white cells. For this reason, injection of insulin into this heterogeneous matrix normally results in a large variation in absorption patterns, even with soluble insulins.[16] Depending upon how the rate of absorption is calculated (e.g. time to maximum peak, concentration at maximum peak, maximal duration, area under the insulin absorption curve), a 50% day-to-day variability is frequently encountered. Furthermore, for complex reasons, only 50% of subcutaneously injected insulin may reach the bloodstream.[17] Consequently, abnormal subcutaneous absorption of insulin is difficult to define unless it is grossly different from the expected variability of normal insulin absorption.

The second reason that subcutaneous tissue is a poor anatomical site to inject insulin is that the blood flow to this tissue is dependent upon many variables.[16] The rate of insulin absorption is greatly affected by the rate of blood flow to the skin, increasing with increasing temperature and decreasing when blood flow is restricted as the temperature of the extremity declines. Blood flow is also altered by the local metabolic needs of the site. For example, an exercising extremity requires increased delivery of nutrients, with the subsequent increased blood flow increasing subcutaneous insulin absorption. This change in blood flow may or may not coincide with the insulin requirements of the diabetic individual. Although the abdomen (as an injection site) compensates for many of these variables, it has its own limitations, such as limited area, tendency for scar formation from surgical interventions and difficult access during social interactions.

The answer to the question of when subcutaneous insulin resistance exists under normal circumstances is 'almost never'.[18] It is conceivable that there may be large areas of scar tissues that are extremely poorly vascularized, so that normal insulin absorption is not possible. In addition, there may be areas of necrotic tissue in which insulin absorption is not possible. In general, however, all tissues demonstrate insulin absorption, although there is significant variability between anatomical sites.

What are alternative interpretations for the clinical reports of subcutaneous insulin resistance?

The subcutaneous tissue contains proteases that can hydrolyse insulin in vitro. Duckworth and colleagues have defined the kinetics of these enzymes when incubated with insulin.[19,20] In a well-characterized patient with increased insulin-degrading activity in the subcutaneous tissue, these authors demonstrated that adipose tissue extracts degraded insulin at a rate of six times that of controls.[1] However, this patient also had increased degradation activity in her serum and required excessive doses of intravenous insulin to maintain metabolic control. Therefore, systemic degradation of insulin was also present. Even individuals with very high levels of subcutaneous degradation activity should demonstrate a measurable quantity of circulating insulin following subcutaneous injection. This is an important concept, since some of the patients originally reported with the syndrome of subcutaneous insulin resistance demonstrated no rise in free insulin concentration following subcutaneous injection. The most obvious conclusion for this observation is that these individuals never received the 'injected' insulin.

Our diabetes centre has received over 30 referrals from physicians throughout the world requesting a second opinion for patients with the presumptive diagnosis of subcutaneous insulin resistance (Table 5.1). In every· instance these referred patients have responded to subcutaneously injected insulin when the insulin (obtained from an unopened bottle) was injected by a physician. The testing needs to be done under rigorously controlled conditions in which the patient has no role in the insulin administration. The details of this testing procedure have been described in detail and the reader is referred to this publication.[18] Briefly, testing for subcutaneous insulin resistance involves giving a standard dose of insulin both subcutaneously and intravenously and comparing the free insulin response to that observed in non-diabetic individuals. We recommend giving 0.5 mg/kg subcutaneously as an initial screen (Fig. 5.1). It is very important that the patient be fasting and well-hydrated; otherwise, the food intake will obscure the hypoglycaemic effect of the insulin. The physician should obtain a new bottle of soluble (regular) insulin from the pharmacy and draw up the insulin in the syringe himself. He should also inject it and permit neither the patient nor the nurse to inject it. This approach may seem overly cautious, but we have observed patients squirting the insulin out of the syringe before injection and substituting water for the insulin in a previously opened vial. Plasma samples for free insulin measurement should be kept at room temperature until insulin antibodies are precipitated with polyethylene glycol (PEG). When such a rigorous testing procedure was followed, we were not able to confirm any patient as having subcutaneous insulin resistance.

If all referral patients responded to subcutaneously injected insulin with a significant increase in circulating plasma free insulin levels, what alternative explanation can be given for their unstable diabetes? As might be anticipated, there is not one simple answer. Extensive investigation and psychological testing are required to determine the underlying cause of the patient's poorly controlled diabetes.[21]

Table 5.1 Long-term follow-up of patients with incapacitating, unstable diabetes

Patient	Aetiology of brittle diabetes	Additional diagnoses or characteristics
1	Factitious disease	Drug addiction
2	Factitious disease	Depression
3	Factitious disease	Superior intelligence
4	Factitious disease	Pathological behaviour
5	Factitious disease	Recurrent sepsis, factitious bleeding diathesis
6	Factitious disease	Obesity
7	Factitious disease	–
8	Factitious disease	Depression
9	Malingering	–
10	.Malingering	School phobia
11	Malingering	Disease denial
12	Malingering	Spouse manipulation
13	Malingering	School phobia
14	Malingering	Spouse manipulation
15	Malingering	School phobia
16	Malingering	Pragmatic language disorder
Communicative disorders		
17	Receptive plus expressive language deficits	Low intellectual functioning
18	Receptive language deficits	–
19	Auditory processing deficits	–
20	Receptive plus expressive language deficits	Pragmatic language disorder
21	Receptive language deficits	Depression
22	Receptive language deficits	–
23	Receptive language deficits	Pragmatic language disorder
24	Diabetic gastroparesis	Depression
25	Diabetic gastroparesis	Depression
Insulin resistance		
26	Systemic	Systemic lupus erythematosus
27	Systemic	Memory and auditory processing deficits
Miscellaneous		
28	Drug addiction	Depression
29	Seizure disorder	Memory deficit
30	Undiagnosed	Insulin allergy

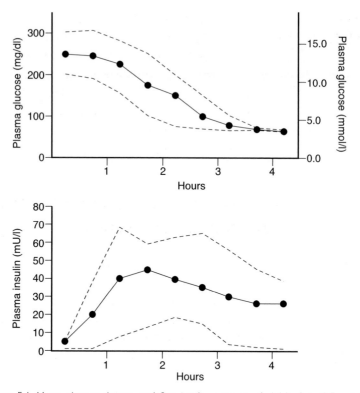

Figure 5.1 *Mean plasma glucose and free insulin responses (solid line) to 0.5 units/kg of subcutaneously injected soluble insulin in 16 unstable diabetic patients referred with the diagnosis of subcutaneous insulin resistance. Note the wide range of responses (±2 SD) in 11 matched control subjects with type 1 diabetes (dotted lines). All referred patients responded to injected insulin when given under rigidly controlled clinical conditions. See reference 18 for additional details.*

However, with perseverance and long-term follow-up, a rational explanation has become evident (Table 5.1).[22] The three most common diagnoses which account for patients given the presumptive diagnosis of subcutaneous insulin resistance are:

- learning disabilities
- manipulative behaviour
- factitious disease.[22]

Other causes, such as undiagnosed drug addiction and severe psychological stress, are uncommon and usually identified by the patient's physician. Manipulative behaviour and factitious disease have been encountered by most physicians and will be briefly described below as a cause of unstable diabetes. However, because learning disabilities are a common cause of unstable diabetes and rarely considered by physicians, the majority of this chapter will provide a short overview of this diagnostic category.

How does manipulative behaviour differ from factitious disease?

The terms 'manipulative behaviour' and 'factitious disease' are often used interchangeably by physicians for patients with unstable diabetes. This is a serious mistake for two reasons: first, the aetiologies of these two entities are different; secondly, the treatment is dependent on the specific diagnosis. Manipulative behaviour always involves a specific goal of the patient, usually to avoid an unpleasant home or work environment. Individuals with this condition learn to use their diabetes to deal with the stresses in their lives. In contrast, factitious disease is behaviour that leads to unstable diabetes but does not have an identifiable rational goal. Why the diabetic patient is performing self-destructive acts to intentionally destabilize their diabetes is not comprehensible to the health care team. In our experience, diabetic patients with unstable diabetes due to manipulative behaviour are frequently female teenagers who are unable to cope with the stresses of school or a poor home environment. They quickly learn that hospitalization for diabetic ketoacidosis removes them from these emotional stresses and places them in a friendly, supportive hospital setting. In contrast, patients exhibiting factitious disease present at all ages with equal sex representation. The one characteristic we have observed in these individuals is above normal intelligence.[22] This is important, since without it the health care team would rapidly identify their factitious behaviour.

Unstable diabetes secondary to manipulative behaviour can be identified by carefully investigating the home and school environment. Interviews with the family members are essential, as well as examining the hospital setting into which these individuals are admitted following metabolic decomposition. These individuals usually have a large group of sympathetic friends (usually the nurses) on the hospital wards and are frequently given privileges not afforded most patients. For example, several of our referred teenage patients had assumed hospital ward clerk duties while recovering from diabetic ketoacidosis. Treatment of these individuals should involve a child psychologist or other professional who has expertise in teenage behaviour. Treatment of this cause of unstable diabetes is usually very successful, either because the hospital environment is made less attractive (e.g. visitors are restricted to parents only) or the patient matures and identifies other strategies to deal with life stresses.

In contrast, factitious behaviour is very difficult to diagnose and treat and may result in an undesirable outcome, including death. It has frequently required months of observation to reach the correct diagnosis in these patients. The factitious diabetic patient is very careful not to perform the self-destructive acts while being observed and is very careful not to leave evidence of her activities. The most important approach for the physician to take is to at least suspect factitious disease in an unstable diabetic patient when no rational cause of the instability is identifiable. Physicians who have referred their patients to us with subcutaneous insulin resistance rarely believe that their patient has factitious disease. Physicians, by the very nature of their training, are taught to believe what their patients report. Treatment of these individuals is usually unsuccessful because the underlying rationale for their behaviour is not understood. Referral to a psychiatrist is always recommended in the medical literature but there is no credible evidence that this alters the natural history of the condition. In our experience, confrontation is also unrewarding, as the patient will change their medical care to another unsuspecting physician. The primary reason to identify this cause of unstable diabetes is to alert the hospital medical staff in order to avoid unnecessary invasive diagnostic procedures that may endanger the life of the patient.

What are learning disabilities and why do they cause unstable diabetes?

Self-management of diabetes requires many abilities: awareness, attention, auditory processing, visual processing, memory, problem solving, reasoning, calculation, information processing, script knowledge, communication, social skills and metacognitive skills. Integration must occur to optimize and maintain glycaemic control. Several conditions in and of themselves create barriers to control. Learning disabilities may preclude the acquisition of necessary skills and result in repeated errors and regimen failures. Advanced disease and prolonged instability may result in complications or cumulative effects that can impair cognition or confer additional risk for error (e.g. hypertension, retinopathy and atherosclerosis). Advancing age may also present problems, including medical and cognitive issues (e.g. mild cognitive impairment, dementia, stroke and polypharmacy). Early identification of problems may thwart repeated failure and unwanted consequences. It can also be expected to minimize the medical, psychological and interpersonal effects of poor control. A community-based, multidisciplinary approach that provides an opportunity for open communication and feedback is the best long-term option. However, identification of the problem is essential to direct referral to appropriate professionals. Failure to define the aetiology of individual treatment failures can lead to social isolation and compound the problem, thereby further reducing the potential for effective care. Working within and around neurobiological constraints is challenging and requires creativity.

Learning disabilities are a heterogeneous group of disorders that can manifest in different ways. Some are severe and others are subtle and emerge in response to heightened levels of (situational) demand. Aetiologies include neurophysiological, genetic, medical, perinatal and environmental factors. Demoralization, poor self-esteem and impaired social skills may accompany a learning disability. The course varies across individuals and may persist across domains. Disorders that involve the processing of information include central auditory processing, visual processing, deficits in selective attention and concentration, memory (retrieval, visual and auditory) and executive abilities involved in organizing and sequencing information. Language disability accounts for a considerable proportion of learning problems observed across academic domains, such as reading (dyslexia), spelling, writing (dysgraphia), language (expressive, receptive), mathematics (dyscalculia, problem solving) and social skills (pragmatic language).

Learning disabilities should be viewed independently of other conditions, and in particular they are not the result of other handicapping conditions such as sensory or motor impairment, mental retardation, social or emotional disturbance, or environmental influences. They are presumed to result from central nervous system dysfunction. Additional problems include the non-verbal domains (coordination, visual–spatial, visual perception, coordination, social perception/competence, emotional maturity). For the individual with a learning disability there is a discrepancy between intellectual potential and academic abilities. Learning disabilities are persistent and continue throughout life, although adaptation and compensatory strategies may render them less problematic over time. For some, failure to address information processing and communication issues results in social as well as educational problems.[23]

An understanding of common difficulties encountered by people with learning disabilities may be helpful for the primary clinician or health care team responsible for diabetes education. This knowledge may result in programme adaptation or alternative methods of teaching. Supplemental materials can be developed through an understanding of issues causing a functional breakdown associated with the management of diabetes. Each learning disability presents the potential for regimen errors, the nature of which are dependent upon the specific disability. This may be important for patient–provider communication when addressing compliance. Selected learning disabilities will be discussed in brief with a discussion of errors that characterize the population in general terms, as there is considerable individual variation.

Individuals with a *reading disability* often make errors characterized by reversals, transpositions, inversions and omissions. Among the problems this can create for someone with diabetes are logging accurate entries into a diary. A *mathematics disability* is generally characterized by difficulty recognizing numbers and symbols, memorizing facts, aligning numbers and understanding abstract concepts. Additionally, there may be impaired visual spatial skills, poor mathematical reasoning and problems in calculation (arithmetic). Monitoring and adjusting for blood glucose levels may be a problem for someone with a maths disability. Another problem that may contribute to medical adherence issues is a disability in the area of *expressive language*, specifically writing. There may be aversion to keeping a log due to problems with grammar, spelling, punctuation and general organization of written material. It is not uncommon to have associated eye–hand coordination problems (absent gross motor problems) and sensory-integration problems. *Receptive language* disorders may result in difficulties in comprehension, processing information, following a conversation, note taking and social relationships. Many of these learning disabilities occur together. Non-verbal learning disabilities, as observed with the language-based disabilities, may also present problems for developing and sustaining good diabetes care. A *non-verbal disability* is characterized by problems in mathematics, spatial orientation, problem solving, motor coordination and social relationships. Impaired kinaesthetic processing and spatial perceptions can create difficulty in responding to novel situations and meeting situational demands. This disorder may interfere with diabetes care in several ways, particularly coping with unanticipated events and the need for structure. Attention disorders are common co-morbidities to the above disorders, further compounding the problem. Although *attention deficit disorder* is not a learning disability per se, it can be expected to negatively influence learning and is characterized by difficulty sustaining attention, attending to details, organizing and sequencing activities, listening, forgetfulness, restlessness, monitoring behaviour and impulse control. The most perplexing of all learning disabilities are individuals who are *gifted with a learning disability* referred to as the 'twice exceptional'. This group, in particular, may be misperceived as non-compliant, given the nature of the disorder.

If a learning disability is suspected, a referral should be made to an appropriate professional (Fig. 5.2). Evaluation may be possible through different agencies if the patient qualifies. Early interventions (educational and psychosocial) have good outcomes. Modifications within the diabetes clinic could also be implemented. These might include individ-

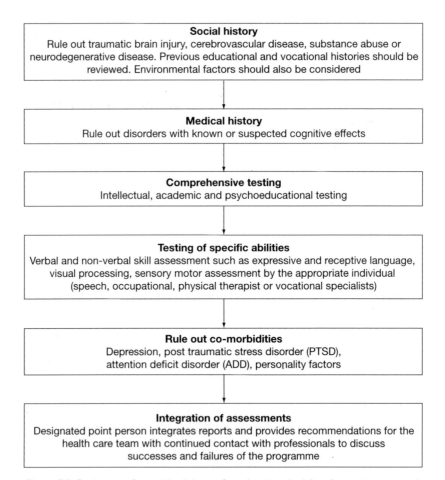

Social history
Rule out traumatic brain injury, cerebrovascular disease, substance abuse or neurodegenerative disease. Previous educational and vocational histories should be reviewed. Environmental factors should also be considered

Medical history
Rule out disorders with known or suspected cognitive effects

Comprehensive testing
Intellectual, academic and psychoeducational testing

Testing of specific abilities
Verbal and non-verbal skill assessment such as expressive and receptive language, visual processing, sensory motor assessment by the appropriate individual (speech, occupational, physical therapist or vocational specialists)

Rule out co-morbidities
Depression, post traumatic stress disorder (PTSD), attention deficit disorder (ADD), personality factors

Integration of assessments
Designated point person integrates reports and provides recommendations for the health care team with continued contact with professionals to discuss successes and failures of the programme

Figure 5.2 *Evaluation of unstable diabetes for a learning disability. A stepwise approach is recommended.*

ual instruction, decomposition of learning into smaller steps, additional time provided for initial presentation of material, multi-modal instruction (visual, auditory, tactile) and supervised practice with immediate feedback. Given that errors result in learning problems, knowledge from one teaching session may not be generalized to the next or to other situations. Therefore, exposure to alternative situations that are commonly experienced by persons with diabetes may be useful.

It is important for the diabetes educator to alter expectations for individuals with learning differences regarding self-care. It must be assumed that they will require additional time, effort and novelty in approach. Creativity will be needed, as will consultation with professionals who have expertise in these areas. Programmes are available for all ages. Adolescents and young adults may benefit from exposure to vignettes related to diabetes-related self-management problems to facilitate problem solving.[24] A 6-week diabetes problem-solving programme for adolescents was found to improve metabolic control, as demonstrated by improved Hb1Ac values and more frequent blood glucose testing, which was maintained for at least 6 months post programme.[25] For older individuals, coaching interventions such as those developed for the purpose of promoting dietary and exercise lifestyle changes for type 2 diabetes – employing educational reinforcement, psychosocial support and motivational guidance – may be beneficial.[26] The support provided by these and similar programmes make available an external structure with successive approximations towards control as skills develop.

What is the current status of subcutaneous insulin resistance as a pathogenic mechanism for unstable diabetes?

From the above discussion, it is reasonable to ask, 'Does the subcutaneous insulin resistance syndrome really exist?' This is a difficult question because it is impossible to prove that it does not. Several lines of evidence, however, suggest that it is extremely unlikely. First, no rational pathogenic mechanism has been suggested which would result in completely absent insulin absorption following subcutaneous injection of insulin. Secondly, no valid case of subcutaneous insulin resistance has been published in which rigid diagnostic guidelines in a controlled setting have been followed to establish the diagnosis. Thirdly, all cases of subcutaneous insulin resistance referred to our centre for a second opinion have been demonstrated to be due to another cause. And fourthly, the frequency of reported cases of subcutaneous insulin resistance, since we published strict diagnostic guidelines, has declined dramatically. However, it is important for investigators to keep an open mind on the possibility that this syndrome may exist.

Conclusions

Subcutaneous insulin resistance implies that insulin is excessively degraded in the subcutaneous tissue, but not excessively destroyed by peripheral tissues such as the liver and kidney. Using this syndrome as a cause of unstable diabetes is problematic because of the great variability of subcutaneous insulin absorption in normal individuals. Attentive causes of unstable diabetes are much more likely and require the physician to perform a careful work-up to identify the correct cause. In our large referral population of unstable diabetes patients, we have not been able to identify one valid case of subcutaneous insulin resistance. Alternative explanations for the metabolic instability include factitious disease, manipulative behaviour and learning disability. The latter category is rarely considered by physicians but constitutes a significant cause of unstable diabetes. Of all the causes of unstable diabetes, these are the most amenable to treatment. Subcutaneous insulin resistance should only be considered when all other causes of unstable diabetes have been excluded.

References

1. Paulsen EP, Courtney JW, Duckworth WC. Insulin resistance caused by massive degradation of subcutaneous insulin. Diabetes 1979; 28: 640–5.
2. Elving LD, Casparie AF, Miedema K, Russchen CJ. Subcutaneous degradation of insulin. Diabetologia 1981; 21: 161–2.
3. Berger M, Halban PA, Girardier L et al. Absorption kinetics of subcutaneously injected insulin: evidence for degradation at the injection site. Diabetologia 1979; 17: 97–9.
4. Maberley GF, Wait GA, Kilpatrick JA et al. Evidence for insulin degradation by muscle and fat tissue in an insulin resistant diabetic patient. Diabetologia 1982; 23: 333–6.
5. Henry DA, Lowe JM, Citrin D, Manderson WG. Defective absorption of injected insulin. Lancet 1978; 2: 741.
6. Muller WA, Tallens C, Lereret S et al. Resistance against subcutaneous insulin successfully managed with aprotinin. Lancet 1980; 1: 1245–6.
7. McElduff A, Eastman CJ, Haynes SP, Bowen KM. Apparent insulin resistance due to abnormal enzymatic insulin degradation: a new mechanism for insulin resistance. Aust NZ J Med 1980; 10: 56–61.
8. Freidenberg GR, White N, Cataland S et al. Diabetes responsive to intravenous but not subcutaneous insulin: effectiveness of aprotinin. N Engl J Med 1981; 305: 363–8.
9. Blazar BR, Whitley CB, Kitabchi AE et al. In vivo chloroquine-induced inhibition of insulin degradation in a diabetic patient with severe insulin resistance. Diabetes 1984: 33: 1133–7.
10. Misbin RI, Almira EC, Cleman MW. Insulin degradation in serum of a patient with apparent insulin resistance. J Clin Endocrinol Metab 1981; 52: 177–80.
11. Campbell IW, Kritz H, Najemnik C, Hagmuller G, Irsigler K. Treatment of type I diabetic with subcutaneous insulin resistance by totally implantable insulin infusion device ("Infusaid"). Diabetes Res 1984; 1: 83–8.
12. Pickup JC, Home PD, Bilous RW, Keen H, Albert KGMM. Management of severely brittle diabetes by continuous subcutaneous and intramuscular insulin infusions: evidence for a defect in subcutaneous insulin absorption. Br Med J 1981; 282: 347–50.
13. Schade DS, Eaton RP, Warhol RM, Gregory JA, Doberneck RC. Subcutaneous peritoneal access device for Type I diabetic patients nonresponsive to subcutaneous insulin. Diabetes 1982; 31: 470–3.
14. Williams G, Pickup JC, Bowcock S, Cooke E, Keen H. Subcutaneous aprotinin causes local hyperaemia: a possible mechanism by which aprotinin improves control in some diabetic patients. Diabetologia 1983; 24: 91–4.
15. Pickup JC, Williams G, Bilous RW, Keen H. Diabetes resistant to subcutaneous insulin: effect of aprotinin. N Engl J Med 1981; 305: 1413.

16. Galloway JA, Spradlin CT, Nelson RL et al. Factors influencing the absorption, serum insulin concentration, and blood glucose responses after injections of regular insulin and various insulin mixtures. Diabetes Care 1981; 4: 366–76.

17. Nelson RL, Galloway JA, Wentworth SM, Caras JA. The bioavailability, pharmacokinetics, and time action of regular and modified insulins in normal subjects. Diabetes 1976; 25(suppl 1): 325.

18. Schade DS, Duckworth WC. In search of the subcutaneous-insulin-resistance syndrome. New Engl J Med 1986; 315: 147–53.

19. Duckworth WC, Gifford D, Kitabchi AE, Ruyan K, Soloman SS. Insulin binding and degradation by muscles from streptozotocin-diabetic rats. Diabetes 1979; 28: 746–8.

20. Duckworth WC, Kitabchi AE. Insulin metabolism and degradation. Endocrinol Rev 1981; 2: 210–33.

21. Schade DS, Drumm DA, Duckworth WC, Eaton RP. The etiology of incapacitating, brittle diabetes. Diabetes Care 1985; 8: 12–20.

22. Schade DS, Drumm DA, Eaton RP, Sterling WA. Factitious brittle diabetes mellitus. Am J Med 1985; 78: 777–84.

23. Cave LJ (Ed). Learning Disabilities, U.S. Department of Health and Human Services, Public Health Service, National Institutes of Health, NIH#93-3611, 1999.

24. Cook S, Aikens JE, Berry CA, McNabb WL. Development of diabetes problem-solving measure for adolescents. Diabet Educ 2001, 27: 865–74.

25. Cook S, Herold K, Edidin DV, Briars R. Increasing problem solving in adolescents with type 1 diabetes: the choices diabetes program. Diabet Educ 2002; 28: 115–24.

26. Whittemore S, Chase S, Mandle CL, Roy SC. The content, integrity, and efficacy of a nurse coaching intervention in type 2 diabetes. Diabet Educ 2001; 27: 887–98.

chapter 6

Psychological factors and glycaemic control

Moyyaad Kamali and Elspeth Guthrie

Introduction

Diabetes is a chronic and disabling illness which affects about 1% of the population. Although most people with diabetes cope well with the condition, psychological problems are common. Such problems are important not only because of the suffering they cause in their own right but also because of their impact on the management and eventual outcome of the diabetes itself. This chapter will focus initially on the psychological adjustment to diabetes, and will then consider the associated specific psychiatric conditions that can occur in relation to the disorder.

Self-care behaviour and blood glucose control

Good self-care and optimal glycaemic control determines the long-term risk of serious medical complications from diabetes. Thus, much closer control over diet, weight and self-care is necessary for people with diabetes than others. However, such rigid control is not easy.

Behaviour that would be considered within the normal range in people without diabetes can appear reckless in those with the condition. Research findings have shown that individuals who tend to lead an ordered existence and have a heightened overall sense of control achieve better metabolic control of their diabetes than those individuals who are more chaotic and disorganized.[1] Feeling in control of other aspects of life, in particular interpersonal relationships and career, are also related to HbA_{1c} status.

Motivation may be an important additional factor determining overall diabetic control,[2] and new psychological techniques involving motivational interviewing are currently being tested to determine their usefulness in promoting better diabetic control.

Psychosocial factors have been shown to affect metabolic control either via neuroendocrine effects or indirectly by influencing patient compliance.[3] It is difficult to adhere to a strict dietary regime or follow medical advice, if one is living in hardship or under severe stress. Psychiatric conditions, such as depression (see later), lead to alterations in mood state and cognitive appraisal that can interfere with adherence. Even relatively mild psychiatric conditions – so called subthreshold states – can have a profound influence on self-care behaviour.

Coping with illness

Physical illness is associated with worry and uncertainty. People react differently to illness, and there is a wide range of normal responses. Coping with illness is a dynamic process that changes over time. People need to manage the initial emotional shock of diagnosis, assimilate information, construct an understanding of the illness, and the limitations or the demands it imposes upon them and formulate ways to cope.

The best determinant of how an individual will cope with an illness is related to his perception of the illness rather than the illness itself. Thus, two people with the same illness, of similar severity, can react very differently, if their perception of the illness differs. If an illness is perceived as being highly threatening, some individuals can respond by denial. In diabetes, this can have a catastrophic effect on later health.

In later stages of the disease, if complications have developed, individuals may have to continue to adjust to a series of problems (e.g. an amputation or failing eyesight) that occur sequentially. This can be very difficult from a psychological perspective, as a further complication can occur before the individual has had time to adjust emotionally to a prior difficulty.

There is some evidence that patients with diabetic complications have more psychological symptoms than those without complications. For example, diabetic people with chronic foot ulceration or a lower limb amputation have higher rates of psychological morbidity and poorer psychological adjustment to illness than people with diabetes with no complications.[4] Interestingly, lower limb amputees have better psycho-social functioning than those diabetics with chronic foot ulceration, some of whom develop a negative attitude to self care of their feet.[5]

Problem solving

People respond and cope differently to different challenges. Success-ful coping involves the capacity to deal with and solve problems effectively. There are two major components of problem solving: problem orientation and problem-solving skills.[6] Both aspects are summarized in Table 6.1.

Chronic disease can be construed as a series of challenges or problems that have to be managed. A recent study of social problem-solving skills in 259 persons with diabetes suggested that there were four different groups: ideal problem solvers; distressed and unskilled problem solvers; pessimistic and frustrated problem solvers; and low-key and managing problem solvers (Table 6.2).[7] There was no differ-ence between the groups in terms of age, gender, type of diabetes or level of education. The majority of people with diabetes fell into the 'ideal problem solving group' or the 'low key and managing

Table 6.1 Problem-solving domains

Problem orientation
Ward off negative emotions (e.g. anger, depression in
  problem-solving situations)
Facilitate positive aspect and a sense of competency
Inhibit tendencies to react impulsively or carelessly
Motivation towards effective problem solving

Problem-solving skills
Definition and identification of main problem
Generation of possible alternative strategies to deal with
  problem
Decide on solution
Implement and monitor problem-solving strategies

group'. Both of these groups reported better adjustment to the illness
than the other two groups. People in the 'distressed and unskilled
group' reported high rates of depression and poor adjustment to their
illness. Their chosen methods of problem solving, such as recklessness, resulting in greater likelihood of complications.

The patient–provider relationship

It is increasingly being recognized that a collaborative relationship
between patient and provider may improve patient adherence and
outcomes in chronic medical illnesses.[8] Researchers have shown that
satisfaction with the interpersonal quality of the patient–provider
relationship is significantly associated with adherence to treatment in
diabetes.[9] A secure attachment style is also important.

Attachment theory proposes that human beings require stable and
secure relationships during infancy and childhood in order to develop

Table 6.2 Different groups of problem solvers in people with diabetes (from reference 7)

Ideal problem solvers
Confident and optimistic approach towards solving problems, unencumbered by negative moods or self-doubt. Employ a wide range of rational problem-solving skills and do not use ineffective strategies (e.g. recklessness or impulsivity)

Distressed and unskilled problem solvers
Negative orientation towards problem solving. Limited number of rational problem solving skills. Tendency to avoid problems or try to solve problems with reckless or impulsive actions

Pessimistic and frustrated problem solvers
Positive orientation towards solving problems, but prone to use ineffectual strategies

Low-key and managing problem solvers
Not motivated to solve problems but not pessimistic in their attitude to problem solving

consistent and supportive ways of relating to others as adults. Individuals internalize earlier experiences with carers and form internal models of whether they are worthy of care themselves (view of self) and whether others can be trusted to provide care (view of others). These internal models, which are sometimes called internal objects, influence the kinds of interactions individuals have with others and their perception of these interactions.

Researchers in North America[10] have shown that individuals with a dismissive attachment style (people who tend to have a positive view of themselves but find it difficult to trust others) have significantly worse glycaemic control than either individuals with a secure attachment (positive view of self and others) or those with a preoccupied attachment

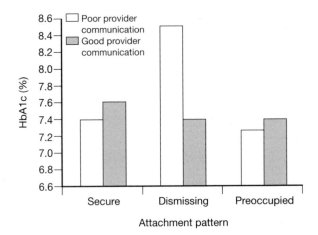

Figure 6.1 *Glycosylated haemoglobin (HbA$_{1c}$) levels of patients with diabetes in relation to attachment category and patient-related quality of provider communication. (Reproduced with kind permission from reference 10.)*

style (negative view of self, but positive view of others) (Fig. 6.1). The investigators suggested that individuals who are highly self-reliant, and find it extremely difficult to trust others, may find it very difficult to form collaborative working relationships with health care professionals.

Of note, within the 'dismissive' group as a whole, those who assessed communication with their doctor/nurse as poor had glycosylated haemoglobin values 1.0% higher than those who assessed their patient–doctor communication as good. The clinical importance of a 1% increase in glycosylated haemoglobin has been demonstrated in one study which showed that such an increase, early in disease, was associated with a nearly 60% increase in the incidence of retinopathy at follow-up.[11]

Depression

Depression is a common illness, associated with significant disability and mortality and it is characterized by low mood and loss of interest

Table 6.3 Common symptoms in depression

Mood and motivation
Low mood (classically worse in the morning)
Loss of interest in normal activities (anhedonia)
Fatigue or loss of energy
Poor concentration
Social withdrawal

Cognitive symptoms
Excessive guilt
Worthlessness
Hopelessness
Suicidal ideation

Physical symptoms
Poor appetite
Weight loss
Sleep disturbance
Decreased sex drive
Retardation or agitation

in usual activities (anhedonia). Low mood can be distinguished from normal sadness by its intensity, duration and pervasiveness. Symptoms of depression can be divided into three categories: mood and motivation, cognitive symptoms and physical symptoms (Table 6.3). The two most widely used diagnostic systems, the DSMIV and the ICD10, require that the symptoms should persist for at least 2 weeks and interfere with normal activities.

A considerable amount of research has shown that individuals with diabetes have a higher risk of developing depression than the general population, with lifetime prevalence rates between 14 and 30% of patients with type 1 or type 2 diabetes, a point prevalence approximately 2–3 times that observed in the general population.[12] The results of a recent meta-analysis of 42 studies of depression in diabetes (20 of which included a non-diabetic control group) has confirmed that there is no difference in the prevalence rates between types 1 or 2 diabetes.[13] In the controlled studies the odds of depression in the diabetic group were twice that of the non-diabetic group. The prevalence of depression was significantly higher in diabetic women (28%) than men (18%) and it was higher in clinical populations (32%) than community samples (30%).

Despite the negative impact of depression on diabetes, it continues to be underdiagnosed, with only one-third of cases recognized and treated in primary care and secondary specialized care.[14] If depression is left untreated, it tends to follow a chronic or relapsing course. An important factor contributing to underdiagnosis is the common assumption that depression in medically ill people is understandable and an acceptable response to a stressful medical illness and not of independent significance.[15] Another problem is that some of the symptoms of depression – e.g. fatigue and anorexia – overlap with symptoms of medical illness. Furthermore, patients' negative attitude to the diagnosis of depression and consequently their unwillingness to report depressive symptoms, as well as the unsuitability of the clinical setting, may play a part.[16]

Depression has been shown to be associated with poorer glycaemic control and raised HbA_{1c} levels in both type 1 and type 2 diabetes.[17] Hyperglycaemia is associated with an earlier onset and progression of diabetic complications, which are linked to poorer quality of life, higher social and vocational impairment and ultimately increased mortality. Worsening mental and physical functioning is associated with increased risk of emergency consultation and inpatient treatment and thus higher direct and indirect health care costs.[18]

Both physiological and behavioural mechanisms have been hypothesized to underly the relationship between depression and glycaemic control. Emotional distress is associated with changes in the sympathetic system and the pituitary–adrenal–cortical axis through the effect of cortisol, as well as increase in glucagon and growth hormone secretion, which are linked to high blood glucose levels.[19] However, behavioural mechanisms are possibly more important: for example, depressive symptoms are associated with less adherence to dietary recommendations and compliance with medical treatment.[12] Negative cognition, which is prevalent in depression, may affect attitude towards self-care strategies such as glucose monitoring and exercise. The direction and mechanism of the association between depression and poor glycaemic control may vary over time, between episodes and between individuals. In a review of the literature, Lustman et al[17] found that in two of three trials of antidepressants in diabetic patients, improvement in depression was associated with improvement in glycaemic control. Conversely, in two trials of oral hypoglycaemic agents, improvement in diabetic control was associated with corresponding improvement in depression. Not only has depression been shown to be related to hyperglycaemia but it also has been shown to be associated with diabetic complications. In a meta-analysis of 27 studies, De Groot et al[20] found a consistently significant association between depressive symptoms and diabetic complications. The effect size was similar across the different complications. Depression may increase the risk of subsequent medical sequelae or, alternatively, complications from diabetes may increase the likelihood of developing depression. Although the direction of causality is not clear, the presence of medical complications early in the course of diabetes should alert physicians to the possibility of depression in this high-risk group of individuals with diabetes.[21]

Assessment of patients with co-morbid depression should include evaluation of suicide risk, psychosocial factors that may contribute to depression as well as considering which treatment is most suitable for a particular individual. Both psychological and pharmacological therapies have been shown to be effective in the treatment of depression in individuals with diabetes. For example, in a randomized controlled trial, 51 patients with diabetes and depression were assigned to a 10-week individual cognitive behavioural therapy (CBT) programme or to a control group. Eighty-five per cent of those who received CBT achieved remission compared to 27% in controls.[22]

Antidepressant medication has also been shown to be effective in the treatment of depressive disorder in individuals with diabetes, but may take 2 weeks and sometimes over 4 weeks before patients can notice any improvement. To improve compliance with medication, it is important that both the patient and physician are aware of the response time. Medication should be continued for 6–9 months after remission of symptoms. Furthermore, prolonged prophylactic antidepressant maintenance is recommended in individuals who experience two or more episodes to prevent relapse. The two most widely used groups of antidepressants are tricyclics and selective serotonin reuptake inhibitors (SSRIs). Tricyclics have been shown to be effective in treating depression in patients with diabetes, although it was associated with hyperglycaemia and disturbed glycaemic control.[23] In addition, tricyclic antidepressants are well recognized for increasing appetite and causing weight gain, which may have a detrimental effect on individuals with diabetes. SSRIs have also been shown to be effective in treating depression in patients with diabetes, and also for improving glycaemic control, probably independent of its effect on mood.[23] This is supported by studies that showed a reduction in HbA_{1c} levels in non-depressed patients with type 2 diabetes.[24] Consequently, SSRIs are preferred to tricyclics as first-line treatment. Some SSRIs can precipitate hypoglycaemic-like episodes in people with diabetes, the mechanism of which is unclear. If this occurs, the patient should be switched to an alternative SSRI. In those individuals who fail to respond to monotherapy, the addition of lithium to an antidepressant or the use of two antidepressants from two different classes can be used, but to date there are no controlled trials to investigate the efficacy of these treatments in depressed patients with diabetes.

Eating disorders

Eating disorders (ED) are not uncommon among adolescents and young adult females in developed countries and there is evidence to suggest that the incidence has increased markedly in recent years, albeit some of the increase being due to greater awareness and reporting of the disorders. There is a 10–20-fold female predominance. Anorexia nervosa (AN) and bulimia nervosa (BN) are the most recognized forms of disordered eating, although subthreshold forms are at least twice as common. AN is characterized by morbid fear of fatness, self-induced weight loss, body image disturbance and the maintenance of weight below that expected for the individual's age, sex and height.

Table 6.4 Diagnosis of eating disorders

Diagnostic criteria for anorexia nervosa (AN):
- Body weight is maintained at least 15% below that expected (for age, sex and height) or body mass index (BMI) is 17.5 or less
- Deliberate weight loss (self-induced vomiting, excessive exercise, abuse of laxatives, appetite suppressant and diuretics and omitting insulin in diabetic patients)
- Morbid fear of fatness and body image distortion. Patients are convinced that they are fat against all evidence to the contrary, even when they are cachectic
- Abnormalities of the hypothalamic–pituitary–gonadal axis, resulting in amenorrhoea in women and loss of sexual interest and potency in men

Diagnostic criteria for bulimia nervosa (BN):
- Morbid fear of fatness
- Preoccupation with eating and craving for food, resulting in bouts of overeating large quantities of food in a short space of time
- Measures to counteract the resultant weight gain from overeating (e.g. self-induced vomiting and purging, intermittent periods of starvation, excessive exercise, use of appetite suppressants and diuretics and omitting insulin in diabetic patients)

BN is distinguished by episodes of overeating or binge eating associated with measures to counteract weight gain. Table 6.4 summarizes the diagnostic guidelines for AN and BN. Apart from the psychopathological aspects of the illness, patients with AN or BN may present with physical or psychological symptoms that are caused by starvation, such as amenorrhoea, hypotension, bradycardia, fatigue, irritability and depression and/or behaviours associated with these syndromes, for example biochemical abnormality as a result of the use of diuretics and laxatives, and dental decay and enlargement of salivary glands as a result of frequent self-induced vomiting.

Studies exploring the prevalence of eating disorders among patients with diabetes have been conducted mainly on patients with type 1 diabetes and have demonstrated inconsistent results. For example, Fairburn and colleagues[25] found no difference in the prevalence of ED in a sample of patients with type 1 diabetes aged 17–25 compared with matched controls of the same age, but he found the underuse of insulin to control weight is widespread and present in over one-third of patients, which was not confined to patients with a clinical eating disorder. Interestingly, none of the men in his study misused insulin to influence their weight. However, Jones et al[26] found that eating disorders and their subthreshold variants are about twice as common in females with type 1 diabetes aged 12–19 compared to age-matched non-diabetic controls, and that ED were associated with an elevated HbA_{1c} level. Researchers have argued that certain features of diabetes, such as dietary restriction associated with treatment and the ability to control the dose or omission of insulin as a method to lose weight, may predispose patients to an eating disorder. Furthermore, the challenge of living with diabetes and its impact on the individual's psychological well-being may also be an aetiological factor.[27] In a study by Steel et al,[28] weight loss at the onset of diabetes and subsequent weight gain with the commencement of insulin was experienced by patients as alarming, and some of the patients developed ED soon after starting treatment.

Although there are conflicting reports regarding the prevalence of ED among patients with diabetes, as pointed out above, there is no argument as to the serious nature of this co-morbidity, coined the 'deadly combination' and 'king of synergism', in which one disorder worsens the other.[27,29] ED have been shown to be associated with poor adherence to diabetic treatment, hyperglycaemia and, consequently, earlier onset of diabetic complications.[30,31] Rydall et al[32] studied 91 young diabetic women at baseline and 4–5 years later and found that 86% and 43% of those with 'highly' and 'moderately' disordered eating behaviour, respectively, had retinopathy compared with only 24% in those without. He reported that disordered eating behaviour accounted for more of the explained variance than did duration of diabetes. Reduction or complete omission of insulin and 'self-induced glycosuria' as a method to reduce weight is reported to be the commonest form of weight control after dieting in most studies. Furthermore, Szmukler[27] noted that the manipulation of insulin is one factor, and that the emotional state associated with ED is another, in causing poor glycaemic control, despite compliance with diabetic regimes.

It is important to identify those with eating disorders before the development of complications and, hence, improve prognosis. Diabetic women with ED may present with less well-recognized features such as treatment non-adherence, poor metabolic control, earlier onset of complications and recurrent ketoacidosis.[32] Consequently, it is important to consider an eating disorder, or at least disturbed eating, in young women with poorly controlled type 1 diabetes. Cantwell and Steel[33] recommended the use of screening tools to identify those at high risk to ensure referral to appropriate services.

Needle phobia

Needle phobia is a marked and persistent fear that is excessive or unreasonable, and provoked by the presence or the anticipation of needles. It is a common fear amongst the general population, with approximately 5–15% refusing necessary dental treatment because of fear of oral injections.[34] Needle phobia can have obvious difficulties for people with diabetes if daily insulin, with associated blood testing, is required. It can also become a serious problem if a person with diabetes has a needle phobia and requires renal dialysis.

Some individuals with needle phobia will refuse to perform any blood glucose monitoring and rely solely upon urine testing to help guide management of their diabetes. Specific phobias are more prevalent in women with type 1 diabetes in comparison with the general population,[35] although the reason for this is unclear. It is possible that sensitization to needles and a conditioning response may occur more frequently in people with diabetes simply because they are more frequently exposed to this noxious experience, in comparison with the general population. There is some evidence that needle phobia runs in families, which may suggest either a genetic contribution or family-learned behaviour.[36]

Treatment usually involves a range of treatment strategies, which are summarized in Table 6.5. Education and reassurance can help the person gain some control over the anxiety associated with needles, and it is important to support self-esteem, as people with this condition can feel silly and ashamed. Physical agents to reduce pain during needle stick procedures can also be helpful. Specific behavioural treatment using psychological desensitization and anxiety management

Table 6.5 Treatment approaches for needle phobia

Education
Reassurance
Maintenance of self-esteem
Pain relief
Anxiety management
Systematic desensitization
Family work to reinforce behavioural treatment
Short-term anxiolytic medication

techniques are the most common forms of psychological intervention. In order for this approach to be successful patients have to be motivated to participate in the treatment, as it involves considerable practice of techniques in between sessions of therapy. Some family interventions may also be necessary to ensure that members of the patient's family do not unwittingly undermine the treatment by seeking to minimize the patient's distress. Short-term low-dose anxiolytic treatment may be considered if a patient's anxiety levels are so high that participation in psychological treatment is hindered. It should never be seen as a stand-alone treatment, because of the risk of dependency.

It is possible that mild needle phobias are quite common in people with diabetes, and they may account for some patient's poor compliance with self-care. Non-invasive monitoring devices may be helpful for such patients, although they are unlikely to be of help for the small number of people with severe needle phobia.

Sexual dysfunction

Diabetes affects sexual function in both men and women, but most studies in the literature are conducted on men and predominantly on erectile dysfunction. This is not surprising, given the high prevalence of the problem among diabetic patients, with reported rates of up to 60%.[37] The prevalence of erectile failure is age-related in the general population[38] and diabetes acts to hasten this process. Interestingly, and counter to common belief, the type of diabetes (whether type 1 or 2) does not appear to influence the development of impotence. However, diabetic control, alcohol consumption, neuropathy and vasculopathy, as well as age, have been reported to predict the development of erectile dysfunction.[39] Other factors may also influence sexual function, such as medication side effects and psychological factors. It has been noted that in the majority of cases erectile failure is the result of the interaction of physical and psychological factors.[40] Psychopathological conditions may be a primary cause of sexual dysfunction or may act to exacerbate any minor organic pathology.

For example, a diabetic man who becomes aware of a decrease in his penile tumescence starts to worry about his ability to perform sexually, resulting in anxiety-induced failure to achieve or maintain erection during intercourse. Unsuccessful experience will increase anxiety further and a perpetual cycle of anxiety and inability to achieve or maintain erection ensues.[41] Performance-anxiety is a common presenting complaint among both diabetic and non-diabetic attendees to psychosexual clinics. Although erectile failure is the commonest and the most widely studied, ejaculatory problems and decrease in sexual desire have also been reported in diabetic patients. For example, in a study by Fairburn et al,[40] half of the patients with diabetes reported ejaculatory disturbance such as absent or retrograde ejaculation, but the commonest problem was 'the absence of the pumping sensation that normally accompanies ejaculation', which was present in over one-third of patients.

Medical assessment of sexual dysfunction should include a thorough medical, interpersonal and psychosocial history, a physical examination and laboratory and specialized tests when required. Special attention should be paid to performance-anxiety, depression and marital disharmony.

Treatment options have improved significantly in recent years, notably since the introduction of Sildenafil (Viagra), which is an orally active selective phosphodiesterase inhibitor that has been shown to improve erectile function by acting on vascular tissue in the penis. It is relatively well tolerated. Headache, flushing and dyspepsia are the commonest side effects. Another oral drug is apomorphine (Uprima), which activates brain dopamine receptors that are involved in penile erection. It is taken as a sublingual tablet. Other treatments include intracavernosal injections (e.g. of papavarine or prostaglandins), vacuum-assisted erection devices, transurethral prostaglandins and surgical procedures such as revascularization and penile prostheses. Psychological management includes treatment of depressive disorder if present with psychotherapy or antidepressants (preferably those with the least sexual side effects). Performance-anxiety is effectively treated using 'Sensate Focus'.[42] This is a treatment programme that contains educational, psychotherapeutic and behavioural elements. Couples are given graded assignments initially to touch and caress each other, except for genitalia, to experience giving and receiving pleasure without being under pressure to 'perform'. This is followed by touching each other, including the genitalia. When each stage is mastered behaviourally and emotionally, they move on to the next stage, aimed at improving erectile function by removing anxiety.

There is a paucity in the literature on the impact of diabetes on the sexual function of women. This may in part be due to the fact that arousal in women is not as essential to sexual intercourse as erection is for men. Furthermore, women may self-medicate with vaginal lubricants without consulting a doctor and some are unaware of the presence of reduced vaginal lubrication. In a recent controlled study of sexual dysfunction in women with type 1 diabetes, Enzlin et al[43] found that diabetic women were significantly more likely to report problems with arousal than controls. The authors also found that diabetic women reported less sexual desire, problems with orgasm, and dyspareunia, but these did not reach statistical significance, possibly due to the small number of participants.

Although some authors have found that sexual dysfunction is related to diabetic complications, others have not,[44] and this issue remains largely unresolved. In a review article, Enzlin et al[45] concluded that although diabetic women may experience decreased sexual desire or pain during intercourse, the main complication is that of impaired arousal with slow or reduced vaginal lubrication. The authors hypothesize that both diabetic men and women are at particular risk of developing problems in the arousal phase of the sexual cycle, presenting as erectile failure in men and slow and/or inadequate lubrication in women.

Summary

Psychological problems and psychiatric illness are more common in people with diabetes than in the general population. The prevalence is similar to other populations of people who suffer from chronic illness.

Depression, eating disorders and anxiety states (such as needle phobias) have been clearly documented in people with diabetes. Even relatively mild psychosocial problems can have serious long-term consequences if they contribute to poor compliance. People with diabetes who are suffering from psychological difficulties require rapid access to psychiatric and psychological help.

References

1. Surgenor LJ, Horn J, Hudson SM et al. Metabolic control and psychological sense of control in women with diabetes mellitus: alternative considerations of the relationship. J Psychosom Res 2000; 49: 267–73.
2. Trigwell PJ, Grant PJ, House AO. Motivation and glycaemic control in diabetes mellitus. J Psychosom Res 1997; 43: 307–15.
3. Helz JW, Templeton B. Evidence for the role of psychosocial factors in diabetes mellitus: a review. Am J Psychiatry 1990; 147: 1275–82.
4. Carrington AL, Mawdsley SKV, Morley M et al. Psychological status of diabetic people with or without lower limb disability. Diabet Res Clin Pract 1996; 32: 19–25.
5. Masson EA, Angle S, Roseman P et al. Diabetic foot ulcers: do patients know how to protect themselves. Pract Diabet 1989; 6: 22–5.
6. D'Zurilla TJ, Nezu A. Problem solving therapy, 2nd edn. Springer, New York, 1999.
7. Elliott TE, Shewchuk RM, Miller DM, Richards JS. Profiles in problem solving: psychological well-being and distress among persons with diabetes mellitus. J Clin Psychol Med Settings 2001; 8: 283–91.
8. Von Korff M, Gruman J, Schaefer J et al. Collaborative management of chronic illness. Ann Intern Med 1997; 127: 1097–102.
9. Sherbourne CD, Hays RD, Ordway L et al. Antecedents of adherence to medical recommendations: results from the Medical Outcomes Study. J Behav Med 1992; 15: 447–68.
10. Ciechanowski PS, Katon WJ, Russo JE, Walker EA. The patient–provider relationship: attachment theory and adherence to treatment in diabetes. Am J Psychiatry 2001; 158: 29–35.
11. Klein R, Klein BE. Relation of glycaemic control to diabetic complications and health outcomes. Diabetes Care 1998; 21(suppl 3): C39–43.
12. De Groot M, Jacobson AM, Samson JA, Welch G. Glycemic control and major depression in patients with type I and type II diabetes mellitus. J Psychosom Res 1999; 46: 425–35.

13. Anderson RJ, Freedland KE, Clouse RE, Lustman PJ. The prevalence of comorbid depression in adults with diabetes: a meta-analysis. Diabetes Care 2001; 24: 1069–78.
14. Lustman PJ, Clouse RE, Griffith LS et al. Screening for depression in diabetes using the Beck Depression Inventory. Psychosom Med 1997; 59: 24–31.
15. Lustman PJ, Griffith LS, Clouse RE et al. Effects of nortriptyline on depression and glucose regulation in diabetes: results of double-blind, placebo-controlled trial. Psychosom Med 1997; 59: 241–50.
16. Peveler R, Carson A, Rodin G. Depression in medical patients. Br Med J 2002; 325: 149–52.
17. Lustman PJ, Anderson RJ, Freedland KE et al. Depression and poor glycemic control: a meta-analytic review of literature. Diabetes Care 2000; 23: 934–42.
18. Ciechanowski PS, Katon WJ, Russo JE. Depression and diabetes: impact of depressive symptoms on adherence, function and costs. Arch Int Med 2000; 160: 3278–85.
19. Kawakami N, Takatusa N, Shimizu H, Ishibashi H. Depressive symptoms and occurrence of type 2 diabetes among Japanese men. Diabetes Care 1999; 22: 1071–6.
20. De Groot M, Anderson RJ, Freedland KE et al. Association of depression and diabetes complications: a meta-analysis. Pychosom Med 2001; 63: 619–30.
21. Peyrot M, Rubin RR. Persistence of depressive symptoms in diabetic adults. Diabetes Care 1999; 22: 448–52.
22. Lustman PJ, Griffith LS, Freedland KE et al. Cognitive behavioural therapy for depression in type 2 diabetes mellitus: a randomised controlled trial. Ann Int Med 1998; 129: 613–21.
23. Goodnick P. Diabetes mellitus and depression: issues in theory and treatment. Psychiat Annals 1997; 27: 353–9.
24. Connolly VM, Gallagher A, Kesson C. A study of fluoxetine in obese elderly patients with type 2 diabetes. Diabet Med 1995; 12: 416–18.
25. Fairburn CG, Peveler RC, Davis B et al. Eating disorder in young adults with insulin dependent diabetes mellitus: a controlled study. Br Med J 1991; 303: 17–20.
26. Jones JM, Lawson ML, Daneman D et al. Eating disorder in adolescent females with and without type 1 diabetes: cross sectional study. Br Med J 2000; 320: 1563–6.
27. Szmukler GI. Anorexia nervosa and bulimia in diabetics. J Psychosom Res 1984; 28: 365–9.
28. Steel JM, Young RJ, Lloyd GG, MacIntyre CCA. Abnormal eating attitude in young insulin-dependent diabetics. Br J Psychiatry 1989; 155: 515–21.
29. Surgenor LJ, Horn J, Hudson SM. Links between psychological sense of control and disturbed eating behaviour in women with diabetes melli-

tus: implications for predictors of metabolic control. J Psychosom Res 2002; 52: 121–8.

30. Steel MJ, Young RJ, Lloyd GG, Clarke BF. Clinically apparent eating disorder in young diabetic women: association with painful neuropathy and other complications. Br Med J 1987; 294: 859–62.

31. Peveler R. Eating disorder and insulin-dependent diabetes. Eur Eat Dis Rev 2000; 8: 164–9.

32. Rydall AC, Rodin GM, Olmsted MP et al. Disordered eating behaviour and the microvascular complications in young women with insulin dependent diabetes mellitus. N Engl J Med 1997; 336: 1849–54.

33. Cantwell R, Steel JM. Screening for eating disorders in diabetes mellitus. J Psychosom Res 1995; 40: 15–20.

34. Lemasney NJ, Holland T, O'Mullane D, O'Sullivan VR. The aetiology and treatment of needle phobia in the young patient – a review. J Ir Dent Assoc 1989; 35: 20–3.

35. Popkins MK, Callies AL, Lentz RD et al. Prevalence of major depression, simple phobia and other psychiatric disorders in patients with long standing type I diabetes mellitus. Arch Gen Psychiatr 1988; 45: 64–8.

36. Kleinknecht RA, Lenz J. Blood/injury fear, fainting and avoidance of medically related situations; a family correspondence study. Behav Res Ther 1989; 27: 537–47.

37. Guirguis WR. Impotence in diabetes: facts and fictions. Diabet Med 1992; 287–9.

38. Feldman HA, Goldstein I, Hatzichristou DG et al. Impotence and its medical and psychosocial correlates: results of the Massachusetts Male Aging study. J Urol 1994; 151: 884–9.

39. McCulloch DK, Young RJ, Prescott RJ et al. The natural history of impotence in diabetic men. Diabetologia 1984; 26: 437–40.

40. Fairburn CG, Wu FCW, McCulloch DK et al. Clinical features of diabetic impotence: a preliminary study. Br J Psychiatry 1982; 140: 447–52.

41. Webster L. Diabetic impotence: pathogenesis and treatment. In: Veves, ed. Contemporary endocrinology: clinical management of diabetic neuropathy. 1996, pp 227–41.

42. Masters WH, Johnson VE. Human sexual inadequacy. Churchill Livingstone, Edinburgh, 1970.

43. Enzlin P, Mathieu C, Van den Bruel A et al. Sexual dysfunction in women with type 1 diabetes. Diabetes Care 2002; 25: 672–7.

44. Tyrer G, Steel JM, Ewing DJ et al. Sexual responsiveness in diabetic women. Diabetologia 1983; 24: 166–71.

45. Enzlin P, Mathieu C, Vanderschueren D, Demyttenaere K. Diabetes mellitus and female sexuality: a review of 25 years' research. Diabet Med 1998; 15: 809–15.

chapter 7

Chronic unstable diabetes and hypoglycaemia

Simon Heller

Introduction

The classical picture of brittle diabetes is of hugely disruptive individuals who demand considerable professional time due to repeated hospital admissions for diabetic ketoacidosis and uncontrolled hyperglycaemia. However, severe unstable diabetes due to hypoglycaemia is probably a greater overall burden both to individuals with diabetes and their family as well as their professional carers. The causes of unstable glycaemic control caused by hypoglycaemia include an obsessive drive to maintain a perfect blood glucose, factitious hypoglycaemia, organic problems such as hypoadrenalism as well as temporary instability following a cluster of hypoglycaemic episodes. It is important for clinicians who have to manage these often difficult cases to have both a good understanding of the pathophysiological processes and a knowledge of the ways in which individuals contribute due to their own behaviour. There are some useful clinical strategies which can help to alleviate and occasionally solve the problem. However, some individuals are subject to recurrent and prolonged episodes which occasionally end in tragedy in the form of death or irreversible cerebral damage. This chapter will survey the epidemiology of brittle diabetes as it pertains to hypoglycaemia, briefly review the physiology and pathophysiology of hypoglycaemia and examine the likely causes of brittle diabetes. Possible management approaches will be considered, before concluding with a discussion of the natural history.

Epidemiology and frequency

It is difficult to obtain an accurate assessment of the proportion of people (Table 7.1) who develop chronic hypoglycaemic instability, in part because of the lack of an agreed definition. There have been few population-based surveys and most research into the problems of hypoglycaemia, including its epidemiology, have taken place in a secondary care setting. Indeed, many studies have been conducted in specialist tertiary referral centres, which, because they tend to attract the most difficult cases, provide a rather distorted view of both the scale of the problem as well as the clinical characteristics of those affected. Furthermore, in the absence of a common definition it is often difficult to decide when the day-to-day difficulties with hypoglycaemia, which affect many people with insulin-treated diabetes, are severe enough to be labelled as chronic instability. Nevertheless, despite these limitations there are sufficient published observational studies to obtain a rough estimate of the scale of the problem.

Gill reported a personal series of 42 severely 'brittle patients' whom he compared to a similar number of stable patients:[1] 86% were relatively young females with a shorter duration of diabetes compared to controls (14 years vs 11 years). Recurrent hypoglycaemia was the main pattern of disease in 12%, whereas an equal proportion had a mixed pattern of instability.

Tattersall et al[2] described the fate of 25 patients with brittle diabetes attending their clinic between 1997 and 1999, of whom 14 had attended the Casualty Department with repeated hypoglycaemia. The

Table 7.1 Reports of chronic glycaemic instability due to hypoglycaemia

Authors	Number (proportion) considered to have hypoglycaemic instability	Age in years (range when identified)	Gender distribution expressed as percentage of females	Nature of survey
Gill[1]	5 (12%)	–	60%	Personal series
Tattersall et al[2]	12 (55%)	–	50%	Clinic population
Gill et al[3,4]	64 (17%)	34 (8–83)	53%	National questionnaire survey
Benbow et al[5]	15 (27%)	70 (60–89)	71%	National questionnaire survey

authors defined hypoglycaemic brittleness as greater than 3 admissions to the Casualty Department in a calendar year, and they concluded that around half of those with 'brittle diabetes' in an unselected population attending secondary care had problems with hypoglycaemia. This figure, which is higher than in other surveys, may have been in part a consequence of the rather broad definition.

In the mid 1990s, Gill et al[3] developed a questionnaire approach to try and estimate the scale and nature of unstable diabetes. They contacted diabetes centres across the United Kingdom and received 315 out of 438 (72%) replies. The prevalence was around 1 per clinic, which translated to approximately 3 per thousand insulin-treated patients. Two-thirds were female, 17% had recurrent hypoglycaemia and 24% mixed instability. In a subsequent paper these 64 individuals were described in more detail.[4] They were generally older (mean age 34 vs 22 years) and there were more males (47%) than the 222 (59%) whose instability was due to hyperglycaemia (92 were reported to have both low and high glucose values as a cause of their brittleness). Psychosocial factors were thought to be responsible in around half the cases, although in contrast to those with repeated DKA, organic factors such as hypoglycaemia unawareness and the effect of alcohol were thought to be significant contributory factors. Three of the 381 were believed to have had a factitious cause for their symptoms. The authors concluded that those with recurrent hypoglycaemia comprised a distinctive subgroup with a different sex and age distribution compared to 'typical brittle diabetes' and a greater contribution from organic causes.

The suggestion that hypoglycaemia is a distinctly different cause of chronic instability than hyperglycaemia also receives support from a further questionnaire survey involving an elderly population.[5] In this study of insulin-treated patients over the age of 60 and who were considered to have lifelong glycaemic instability, 56% of questionnaires were returned. The mean age was 74; 27% were thought to have pure hypoglycaemic 'brittleness' and 50% had a mixed picture. Unlike younger age groups, there were few cases of known factitious disease and the authors suggested that the pattern of disease in this age group was also different, with the implication that hypoglycaemia as a cause of instability was more common in this age group.

These reports suggest that the proportion of those with chronic glycaemic instability caused by hypoglycaemia is around 15–25% of the total. This may amount to a total of between 150 and 250 individuals in the UK. The results for the studies discussed here are summarized in Table 7.1.

The normal counter-regulatory response and its contribution to recognition of hypoglycaemia

In non-diabetic individuals, a series of physiological responses prevent the development of severe hypoglycaemia (Table 7.2) even after a prolonged fast, although transient mild hypoglycaemia down to levels as low as 3.0 mmol/l is not uncommon, particularly during the night. The most important protective mechanism appears to be the complete inhibition of insulin secretion whenever blood glucose falls below 4 mmol/l.[6] However, additional responses, operating to maintain blood glucose, probably reflect the survival advantage of physiological defences which ensure continued fuel delivery to the central nervous system (CNS) when the source of the next meal is uncertain. The need for a constant fuel supply to the brain has resulted in considerable redundancy in the systems that maintain blood glucose and they have proved extremely useful in protecting people with insulin-treated diabetes from hypoglycaemia. This is highlighted by the low rates of severe hypoglycaemia in those with recent onset diabetes whose counter-regulatory defences remain intact.[7] It is in marked contrast to the major problems experienced by some of those with longstanding diabetes or tight metabolic control with impaired protective responses, who are often subject to repeated and severe hypoglycaemic episodes.[7,8]

Table 7.2 Mechanisms which help to protect patients with diabetes from severe hypoglycaemic episodes

- Endogenous insulin secretion (associated with preserved glucagon responses and less erratic insulin profiles)
- Counter-regulatory hormone release:
  glucagon ⎫ the two primary hormones
  adrenaline (epinephrine) ⎭ opposing insulin
  growth hormone
  cortisol
- Sympathoadrenal activation
- Autonomic symptoms:
  tremor
  palpitations
  sweating
- Neuroglycopenic symptoms:
  loss of concentration
  confusion
  altered mood
  bad temper
  blurred vision

An array of hormones oppose the action of insulin, both by inhibiting peripheral uptake of glucose in insulin-sensitive tissues such as fat and muscle and stimulating hepatic glucose release through a combination of glycogenolysis and gluconeogenesis. Glucagon appears to have the most rapid and powerful effect and is considered the major counter-regulatory hormone.[9] If its release is inhibited during experimental studies, then blood glucose recovery is inhibited by around 40%. Glucose recovery then relies upon the activation of the sympathoadrenal system and accompanying adrenaline (epinephrine) secretion. If the release of both adrenaline (epinephrine) and glucagon are prevented pharmacologically, then blood glucose recovery from acute insulin-induced hypoglycaemia is almost completely prevented.[10] However, although this suggests that the release of other counter-regulatory hormones such as cortisol and growth hormone are not relevant to blood glucose recovery, case reports of occasional severe hypoglycaemia in individuals with cortisol or growth hormone deficiency[11] indicate a physiological role perhaps by preventing fasting hypoglycaemia.

The ability of an intact counter-regulatory response to prevent severe hypoglycaemia is demonstrated by experiments in which elevating insulin levels three to four times above normal leads to an initial fall but then stabilization of blood glucose at around 3.0 mmol/l.[12] Furthermore, other features of the sympathoadrenal discharge provide an additional defence for those with diabetes by causing hypoglycaemic symptoms. Activation of the sympathetic nervous system generates symptoms of autonomic activation which alert patients (and often their partners or friends) of the need to treat the episode with food.[13] Insulin-treated patients also develop symptoms due to cerebral dysfunction (neuroglycopenia), such as loss of concentration, altered conscious level, emotional lability and bad temper followed by confusion.[14] Many individuals with insulin-treated diabetes learn to rely on such symptoms, particularly if, as their duration of diabetes increases, the intensity of their autonomic response is reduced. Some patients become adept at identifying the start of hypoglycaemia based on a minor loss of concentration or an inability to focus on a reading or writing task. However, since these symptoms represent a failure of brain function, unless hypoglycaemia is corrected rapidly, blood glucose will continue to fall and cerebral dysfunction will increase to a level which prevents that individual from taking the appropriate corrective action. They will then remain incapacitated until either they are revived by someone else or their glucose returns towards normal levels as the injected insulin is cleared from subcutaneous depots. There is, of course, a risk that such an episode will cause permanent cerebral damage or even death, although in practice such outcomes are extremely rare and recovery is usually complete.

The causes of impaired endocrine counter-regulation and hypoglycaemia unawareness

Long duration and intensified insulin therapy

Counter-regulatory responses are intact at diagnosis but gradually become impaired with increasing duration of diabetes. Of the array of protective mechanisms against hypoglycaemia, the first to decline is the glucagon response. A few individuals exhibit diminished responses within a few weeks[15] of developing diabetes but diminished secretion during hypoglycaemia only becomes common after a diabetes duration of 5 years.[16] After 15 years a severely diminished or absent response is almost universal.[16] The failure of the response does not reflect an inability of the α cell to secrete glucagon, as they respond normally to other stimuli such as arginine.[15] The precise mechanism of the defect is still debated, but emerging evidence suggests that release of glucagon during hypoglycaemia depends upon paracrine communication between α and β cells within the islet.[17,18] Defective glucagon secretion during hypoglycaemia reflects a loss of the endogenous insulin release due to β-cell destruction. The progressive failure of activation of the sympathoadrenal system during hypoglycaemia takes longer but is often impaired in those with a duration of diabetes of over 15 years.[16] The precise mechanism of progressive sympathoadrenal failure during hypoglycaemia is also unknown but may relate to progressive damage (perhaps due to repeated hypoglycaemic episodes) to the glucose-responsive neurones in the hypothalamus which activate the autonomic response.

In addition to increasing duration of diabetes, the other important cause of impaired counter-regulation and loss of awareness is that which follows intensified insulin therapy, particularly when it is accompanied by improved glycaemic control and periods of hypoglycaemia. The reports of impaired physiological defences to hypoglycaemia in tightly controlled patients with type 1 diabetes emerged in the mid 1980s.[19,20] The release of adrenaline (epinephrine) and other counter-regulatory hormones during hypoglycaemia was impaired due to altered glycaemic thresholds.[21] These were activated at a lower blood glucose than normal, with responses occurring at values of around 2.5 mmol/l rather than a normal level of 3.5 mmol/l. In such a situation, cerebral function becomes impaired before the activation of counter-regulatory mechanisms, so by the time peripheral changes such as sweating and tremor begin to appear the individual is often incapacitated and unable to take action to raise their blood glucose.[22]

A reduced ability to recognize the onset of hypoglycaemia (hypoglycaemia unawareness) usually reflects general loss of counter-regulatory mechanisms, including the release of adrenaline (epineph-rine).[13,23] Since such a defect develops in addition to a loss of the glucagon response, those affected lack the two main endocrine defences against insulin-induced hypoglycaemia. In the absence of symptoms such as sweating, tremor and palpitations, they rely on neuroglycopenic symptoms which are unreliable and give them little time to correct their low glucose. When severe, this acquired compli-cation of diabetes is a potentially disastrous situation for those affected and their family. The earliest manifestation of hypoglycaemia experienced by individuals is often when they begin to act abnor-mally, perhaps losing their temper or behaving inappropriately. In the most extreme cases, a family member has to be in almost constant attendance.

Its pathogenesis appears to be a consequence of a resetting of the glycaemic threshold for the release of glucagon, and activation of the autonomic nervous system to a glucose concentration well below that for generalized cerebral dysfunction. It occurs, at least in part, due to repeated episodes of hypoglycaemia[12] which reset the glycaemic threshold for physiological responses to hypoglycaemia[24] possibly due to altered cerebral glucose uptake[25] or perhaps surges in cortisol.[26] The absence of counter-regulatory hormone release at mild hypoglycaemic levels of around 3.0–3.5 mmol/l means that blood glucose falls rapidly to lower blood glucose concentrations, at which point cognitive ability deteriorates.[27] The eventual activation of protective physiological responses, albeit at lower glucose levels (usually at around

2.0–2.5 mmol/l),[23] presumably explains why even in those with apparently complete unawareness, blood glucose eventually stabilizes, even during a severe episode, and does not lead to permanent brain damage.

Causes of hypoglycaemic instability (see Table 7.3)

Temporary instability following a cluster of hypoglycaemic episodes

A common pattern for many patients with type 1 diabetes is that they experience a generally stable level of glycaemic control, but which is punctuated by periods of weeks or sometimes months of suddenly fluctuating levels of glycaemic control characterized by a tendency to repeated hypoglycaemia. Such a period is often precipitated by one or two unusually severe hypoglycaemic attacks or the sudden determination of an individual to improve their glycaemic control, perhaps due

---

Table 7.3 Causes of hypoglycaemic instability

Temporary instability after a cluster of hypoglycaemic episodes
Obsessional pursuit of normoglycaemia
Factitious hypoglycaemia
Organic causes:
    Addison's disease
    hypopituitarism
    diabetic nephropathy
    diabetic gastroparesis
    pregnancy
    chronic pancreatitis
    pancreatectomy
    malabsorption
    alcohol

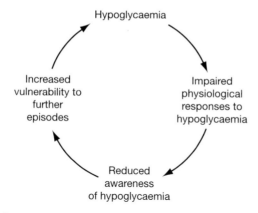

Figure 7.1 *Effect of repeated episodes of hypoglycaemia.*

to a wish to become pregnant or following the discovery of diabetic complications. Patients then go on to develop a 'roller coaster' pattern of blood glucose profiles, with low blood glucose values treated with excessive amounts of glucose or other types of refined carbohydrate. This results in subsequent high values, which are then treated with excessive corrective doses of insulin. The subsequent vulnerability to hypoglycaemia is exacerbated by repeated episodes of hypoglycaemia, which impair endocrine counter-regulation and reduce hypoglycaemic warning symptoms.[28,29] The constant need to correct high and low values soon becomes exhausting and demoralizing for both patient and their partner or family. Such episodes are probably a consequence of a sudden reduction in counter-regulatory hormone protection as a result of one or more episodes of hypoglycaemia itself. This acquired vulnerability to further episodes (Fig. 7.1), coupled with a less-informed approach to maintaining tight glucose control, are probably the main reasons for this pattern of hypoglycaemic instability.

Obsessional pursuit of constant normoglycaemia

Increased duration of diabetes and intensive insulin therapy are common causes of impaired counter-regulation and reduced hypoglycaemia warning symptoms. However, although diminished physiological defences to hypoglycaemia are almost the rule in long-standing type 1 diabetes, only a few patients experience major clinical problems with hypoglycaemia. It is probably a combination of different factors which determine whether those affected go on to develop difficulties with recurrent episodes. In contrast to the problem of hyperglycaemic instability, which is largely due to a failure of the patient to collaborate with their professional carers, many of those who experience problems with hypoglycaemia are in some respects at the opposite end of the spectrum. Most clinicians will be familiar with the obsessional patient who, terrified of tissue complications, maintains blood glucose concentrations at or below 7.0 mmol/l. They often measure their blood glucose many times a day and any value above this narrow range is immediately treated with an extra dose of fast-acting insulin.[30] Unsurprisingly, such individuals are prone to regular and severe hypoglycaemia compounded by a vicious cycle of impaired counter-regulatory hormone responses caused by repeated hypoglycaemic episodes and vulnerability to further attacks. Such patients can be identified by HbA$_{1c}$ values in the non-diabetic range, and although they are often reluctant to admit to their behaviour, family members or friends may reveal the major domestic disruption caused by such an approach.

Factitious hypoglycaemia

In contrast to the conduct of those described above, a rare but distinct group of patients with 'hypoglycaemic brittleness' exhibit factitious behaviour which closely parallels that of those experiencing chronic hyperglycaemic instability. Some publications reporting this phenomenon have classified those affected into two broad groups. Those without diabetes are usually health care workers or individuals with close relatives with diabetes, and have easy access to sulphonylurea drugs or insulin. The other group consists of patients with diabetes. Some fall into the classical picture of the teenage girl with brittle diabetes who presents with either recurrent DKA or severe hypoglycaemia on different occasions. Schade et al, describing their systematic investigation of patients referred with brittle diabetes in the mid

1980s, highlighted the case of a 28-year-old female nurse with type 1 diabetes and a 5-year history of recurrent incapacitating hypoglycaemia, which was always cured by her hospital admission.[31] Hypoglycaemic comas were accompanied by extremely high circulating insulin concentrations. Despite an absence of C-peptide (which excluded an insulinoma), the patient denied taking additional insulin, refused psychiatric help and continued to induce hypoglycaemic seizures.

Grunberger et al reported 10 patients with factitious hypoglycaemia of whom 5, all women, had type 1 diabetes.[32] Three of the five admitted taking excessive insulin and underwent successful psychiatric treatment while of the other two who denied injecting inappropriately, one was found dead 4 months later and the other was lost to follow-up. Two additional cases have been reported by Schuler et al, of whom one was described as 'enjoying' the experience of hypoglycaemia.[33]

Organic causes

Organic causes are relatively uncommon, but once recognized are usually easy to treat. Addison's disease, although rare, occurs more commonly in individuals with type 1 diabetes and usually presents with weight loss and increased frequency of hypoglycaemia. Hardy et al reported two patients who presented with brittle diabetes and severe recurrent hypoglycaemia.[34] Both were found to have glucocorticoid deficiency, one with hypopituitarism and the other with primary adrenal failure. Steroid replacement therapy abolished the hypoglycaemia.

Patients with diabetic nephropathy are also prone to an increased frequency of hypoglycaemia,[35] in part due to a reduction in insulin clearance but also because autonomic neuropathy, common in such patients, leads to irregular absorption of food due to impaired gastric emptying.[36] The first trimester of pregnancy is also associated with a high rate of severe hypoglycaemic episodes.[37] The reasons for this increased vulnerability are not clear. Alterations in gastric emptying and pregnancy-induced vomiting undoubtedly play a part, but it is possible that pregnancy itself may alter the hormonal response to hypoglycaemia and reduce hypoglycaemia awareness.

Diabetes secondary to chronic pancreatitis and following pancreatectomy can be associated with brittle diabetes and a tendency to recurrent hypoglycaemia.[38] Patients are characteristically sensitive to insulin and, although often insulin-requiring, increasing the dose above a few units a day results in recurrent and sometimes severe hypoglycaemic episodes. A number of factors contribute to the increased risks of hypoglycaemia.[39] Damage to islet tissue impairs glucagon production as well as insulin, which increases insulin sensitivity as well as removing one of the primary endocrine defences combating hypoglycaemia. Many patients with pancreatic disease tend to abuse alcohol, which, as described below, increases susceptibility to hypoglycaemia in different ways. Finally, damage to the exocrine pancreas may cause malabsorption and, although this primarily affects fat digestion, any patient with severe malabsorption, particularly if it leads to loss of weight, will become more insulin sensitive and be more vulnerable to hypoglycaemia.

Chronic alcohol ingestion may increase the risk of hypoglycaemia if it leads to chronic pancreatitis, but alcohol has other acute effects which can lead to hypoglycaemia and increase the likelihood of a severe episode, particularly in those who run their blood glucose levels close to normal. Contrary to popular belief, alcohol does not lower blood glucose, but impairs the physiological response to a low blood glucose. Gluconeogenesis is inhibited, perhaps due to a fall in circulating non-esterified fatty acids (NEFAs),[40] and loss of this protective response may increase the severity of a single episode. Alcohol also reduces some of the peripheral autonomic responses (such as tremor) which alert patients to a falling blood glucose.[41] In addition, the neuroglycopenic features of a hypoglycaemic attack such as disinhibited behaviour, confusion or impaired consciousness may be attributed by bystanders to intoxication. Thus, the potential for alcohol to transform moderate hypoglycaemia into a severe episode, or a severe attack into one which results in permanent brain damage or death, is considerable. It is difficult to gauge to what extent alcohol

148

contributes to severe hypoglycaemic episodes overall, but anecdotal reports suggest that it is a common and important factor.[42]

Treatment of common organic causes, approaches to reversing unawareness and enlisting the cooperation of patients (see Fig. 7.2)

Clearly, the priority in responding to hypoglycaemic instability is in identifying the underlying cause. If those affected have an obvious organic precipitant then treatment is straightforward. Thus, standard treatment of conditions such as Addison's disease or hypopituitarism will resolve the problem. Other intercurrent disorders such as impaired renal function are not always as easy to treat. In such patients it is logical to use small amounts of rapid-acting insulin – perhaps with insulin analogues such as lispro or aspart – postprandially.

There is little specific treatment for those experiencing recurrent episodes of hypoglycaemia during pregnancy. It is difficult for those affected to alter their glycaemic targets during the early part of their pregnancy, but there is a tendency for problems with hypoglycaemia to resolve as the pregnancy progresses. Although there has been some debate as to whether rapid-acting insulin analogues are safe to use during pregnancy,[43] they are already used increasingly, particularly for those who are experiencing recurrent and severe nocturnal episodes.[44]

Patients with glycaemic instability related to acquired defects in the physiological response to hypoglycaemia and hypoglycaemia unawareness may respond to an approach which seeks to avoid all episodes of hypoglycaemia, at least in part. Perhaps the most important ingredient is the development of a supportive relationship with a diabetes health care professional – usually a diabetes nurse specialist. The person affected needs to eliminate all episodes of hypoglycaemia, probably for as short a time as 3–4 weeks, to restore some symptomatic awareness.[45,46] Those undertaking such a programme

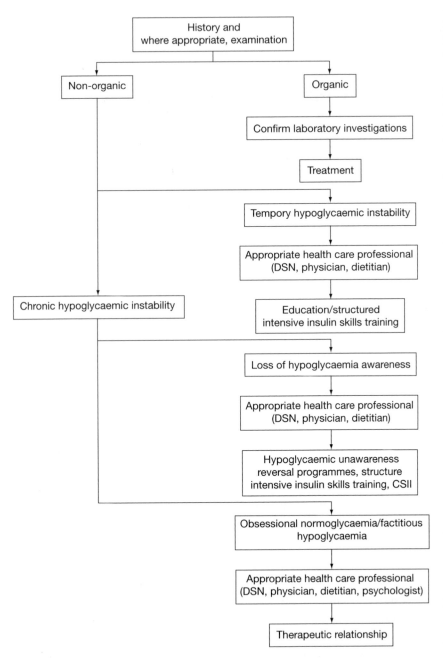

Figure 7.2 *An approach to the patient presenting with hypoglycaemic metabolic instability.*

need to monitor their blood glucose frequently and adjust their insulin to prevent their glucose from falling below normal. They also need to take special precautions during the night, and check their blood glucose between 2 and 3 a.m. It is often difficult to adjust basal insulin to achieve stable overnight glucose levels, although the use of insulin glargine or insulin infusion pumps are being increasingly employed to deal with this particular problem. Most of the published series of successful reversals have not resulted in significant deterioration in HbA_{1c}, although it has tended to rise. It does seem possible to achieve some reversal of unawareness and a fall in frequency of severe hypoglycaemic episodes while still maintaining HbA_{1c} levels in the region of 7–8%. Although the intensity of hypoglycaemic warning symptoms increases, the data surrounding the release of counter-regulatory hormones are less clear. No study has demonstrated restoration of the glucagon response, but two early studies demonstrated recovery of adrenaline (epinephrine) secretion during hypoglycaemia.[45,46] However, a third study reported improved symptomatic responses, although defective counter-regulatory hormone responses were unchanged.[47]

Insulin pump treatment

Although the first studies which used portable infusion pumps to deliver a continuous supply of insulin subcutaneously had suggested that such a system might reduce the risk of hypoglycaemia,[48] early experience of severe episodes during pump therapy seemed to contradict this suggestion.[49] This was reinforced by the Diabetes Control and Complications Trial (DCCT) where rates of severe hypoglycaemia were three times higher in the intensified arm, with no difference between multiple injections and continuous subcutaneous insulin infusion (CSII).[50] However, more recent experience has indicated that pump therapy can reduce the risk of hypoglycaemia in patients aiming for tight glucose control. Bode and colleagues have reported dramatic reductions in the risk of severe hypoglycaemic episodes during a recent trial, with reductions of over 80%.[51] It appears that CSII, which can provide a more reliable and consistent delivery of basal insulin (particularly during the night), has the potential to reduce the risk of hypoglycaemia. It is not entirely clear why the early unfavourable experience has been superseded by more promising results. It may relate in part to a better understanding of how to use the technology to deliver insulin more safely.[52] Alternatively, as described below, the essential elements of pump therapy, which include teaching users to count the carbohydrate content of their meals and then adjust meal-related insulin appropriately, may make an important contribution. The impressive reductions in hypoglycaemia described in recent studies have the potential to maintain or restore some of the components of the physiological defences to hypoglycaemia, although this attractive hypothesis still has to be tested in a formal study.

Specific skills training

In the important studies from Schade and colleagues in the USA, which established that most cases of apparent brittle diabetes were due to lack of patient cooperation or factitious behaviour, they highlighted a small group who they concluded were brittle due to 'communicative' problems.[53] It is difficult to be sure of their exact meaning, but it is increasingly clear that patients who embark on intensive insulin therapy need to have the appropriate self-management skills if they are going to improve their glycaemic control without an epidemic of hypoglycaemia. Berger and Mühlhauser have highlighted the high rates of severe hypoglycaemia during the intensive arm of the DCCT and the major differences between centres,[54] and have suggested that the ability of health care professionals to train patients in intensive insulin therapy may be one of the most important determinants of subsequent hypoglycaemic risks. In a provocative commentary, they proposed that those centres with the highest rates of severe episodes may not have had the skills to train patients to undertake intensive therapy safely.[55] They and others have advocated a structured training package to institute intensive insulin therapy using adult education group techniques, and an approach to eating which encourages dietary freedom and insulin dose adjustment to maintain tight glucose targets.[56-58] The other important component is separation of basal and meal-related insulin. The published data from their group, and those of others following a similar approach, are impressive both in terms of risks of severe hypoglycaemia and glycaemic control,[59] as well as psychological outcomes including treatment satisfaction and quality of life[58] (although there are few randomized controlled trials[60]). Their results suggest that a systematic institution of such an approach has the potential to allow a significant proportion of those with type 1 diabetes to attain glycaemic control comparable to the intensive arm of the DCCT, but with lower rates of severe hypoglycaemia. It is not surprising that this type of approach has considerable similarity to CSII training programmes in which the basal and meal-related components of insulin therapy are also separated, and estimation of carbohydrate intake is important. Indeed, much of the benefit of CSII may well be due to the skills training which necessarily has to be undertaken before patients can safely be supplied with a pump. Other approaches such as blood glucose awareness training (BGAT),[61] which have also been reported to benefit patients experiencing problems with hypogly-caemia, may also owe their success to the skills in self-management acquired by those who participate.

Natural history

Relatively few studies have examined the natural history of chronic unstable diabetes characterized by hypoglycaemia, but those that have indicate important differences in the prognosis of those who present with hypoglycaemic instability compared to those with recurrent hyperglycaemia. Williams and Pickup described 13 patients who had originally been studied in the early 1980s:[62] only one had experienced hypoglycaemic instability, although another 7 had suffered from recurrent episodes of both hyper- and hypoglycaemia. Interestingly, one of the women who had originally presented with episodes of hyper-glycaemia died 2 years later after a prolonged hypoglycaemic attack, which was thought to have been deliberately induced. The authors reported that the majority of patients continued to have problems with unstable diabetes, including those with previous problems of hypoglycaemia, although the severity of their condition had lessened over the years. This may relate to the nature of these referrals, as all were treated in a tertiary referral centre, and it may be that these more severe cases tend to do less well.

Tattersall et al reported the outcome of 25 patients who had originally been reported 15 years before with brittle diabetes:[2] 14 patients had experienced repeated episodes of severe hypoglycaemia of whom 2 had died of uraemia within a year of ascertainment, and a further 2 of hypoglycaemic coma. Five of the 14 patients had continued to experience hypoglycaemic episodes: 2 were thought to have personality disorders and 3 were convinced that their blood glucose should remain below 5.0 mmol/l. Only 3 patients appeared to be prone to hypoglycaemia due to long-standing diabetes and loss of hypoglycaemia awareness. The authors highlighted the poor prognosis of those affected by hypoglycaemic instability (30% mortality over 12 years), although they concluded that even in this group the frequency of admissions declined over time.

Conclusions

Unstable diabetes due to recurrent hypoglycaemia appears to be a distinct category with different causes and presentations, although some patients do present with similar characteristics to those with recurrent hyperglycaemia. The main causes are related to inappropriate behaviour on the part of the patients or their family. If organic causes are considered, they are usually easy to recognize and treat. Encouraging patients to change their behaviour is often difficult, and successful outcomes depend upon the development of a strong therapeutic relationship between those affected and members of the diabetes health care team. There is limited evidence to predict the outlook for those affected, but available data suggest that their prognosis may be worse than those experiencing hyperglycaemia.

References

1. Gill GV. The spectrum of brittle diabetes. J R Soc Med 1992; 85: 259–61.
2. Tattersall RB, Gregory R, Selby C et al. Course of brittle diabetes: 12 year follow up. Br Med J 1991; 302: 1240–3.
3. Gill GV, Lucas S, Kent LA. Prevalence and characteristics of brittle diabetes in Britain. Quart J Med 1996; 89: 839–43.
4. Gill G, Lucas S. Brittle diabetes characterised by recurrent hypoglycaemia. Diabet Metab 1999; 25: 308–11.
5. Benbow SJ, Walsh A, Gill GV. Brittle diabetes in the elderly. J R Soc Med 2001; 94: 578–80.
6. Cryer PE. Hierarchy of physiological responses to hypoglycemia: relevance to clinical hypoglycemia in type I (insulin dependent) diabetes mellitus. Horm Metab Res 1997; 29: 92–6.
7. White NH, Skor DA, Cryer PE et al. Identification of type 1 diabetic patients at increased risk for hypoglycemia during intensive therapy. N Engl J Med 1983; 308: 485–91.
8. Gold AE, MacLeod KM, Frier BM. Frequency of severe hypoglycemia in patients with type I (insulin dependent) diabetes with impaired awareness of hypoglycemia. Diabet Care 1994; 17: 697–703.
9. Cryer PE. Glucose counterregulation: the prevention and correction of hypoglycemia in humans. Am J Physiol 1993; 264: E149–55.
10. Rizza RA, Cryer PE, Gerich JE. Role of glucagon, catecholamines, and growth hormone in human glucose counterregulation. J Clin Invest 1979; 64: 62–71.
11. Smallridge RC, Corrigan DF, Thomason AM et al. Hypoglycemia in pregnancy. Occurrence due to adrenocorticotropic hormone and growth hormone deficiency. Arch Intern Med 1980; 140: 564–5.
12. Heller SR, Cryer PE. Hypoinsulinemia is not critical to glucose recovery from hypoglycemia in humans. Am J Physiol 1991; 541–8.
13. Heller SR, Macdonald IA, Herbert M et al. Influence of sympathetic nervous system on hypoglycaemic warning symptoms. Lancet 1987; ii: 359–63.
14. Deary IJ, Hepburn DA, MacLeod KM et al. Partitioning the symptoms of hypoglycaemia using multi-sample confirmatory factor analysis. Diabetologia 1993; 36: 771–7.
15. Gerich JE, Langlois M, Noacco C et al. Lack of glucagon response to hypoglycaemia in diabetes; evidence for an intrinsic pancreatic alpha cell defect. Science 1973; 182: 171–3.
16. Bolli GB, De Feo P, Compagnucci P et al. Abnormal glucose counterregulation in IDDM. Interaction of anti-insulin antibodies and impaired glucagon and epinephrine secretion. Diabetes 1983; 32: 134–41.
17. Peacey SR, Rostami-Hodjegan A, George E et al. The use of tolbutamide-induced hypoglycemia to examine the intraislet role of insulin in

mediating glucagon release in normal humans. J Clin Endocrinol Metab 1997; 82: 1458–61.

18. Banarer S, McGregor VP, Cryer PE. Intraislet hyperinsulinemia prevents the glucagon response to hypoglycemia despite an intact autonomic response. Diabetes 2002; 51: 958–65.

19. Simonson DC, Tamborlane WV, Defronzo RA et al. Intensive insulin therapy reduces counterregulatory hormone responses to hypoglycaemia in patients with type 1 diabetes. Ann Intern Med 1985; 103: 184–90.

20. Amiel SA, Tamborlane WV, Simonson DC et al. Defective glucose counterregulation after strict glycemic control of insulin-dependent diabetes mellitus. N Engl J Med 1987; 316: 1376–83.

21. Amiel SA, Sherwin RS, Simonson DC et al. Effect of intensive insulin therapy on glycemic thresholds for counterregulatory hormone release. Diabetes 1988; 37: 901–7.

22. Heller SR, Macdonald IA. Physiological disturbances in hypoglycaemia: effect on subjective awareness. Clinl Sci 1991; 81: 1–9.

23. Hepburn DA, Patrick AW, Brash HM et al. Hypoglycaemia unawareness in type 1 diabetes: a lower plasma glucose is required to stimulate sympathoadrenal activation. Diabet Med 1991; 8: 934–45.

24. Widom B, Simonson DC. Intermittent hypoglycemia impairs glucose counterregulation. Diabetes 1992; 41: 1597–602.

25. Boyle PJ, Kempers SF, O'Connor AM et al. Brain glucose uptake and unawareness of hypoglycaemia in patients with insulin-dependent diabetes mellitus. N Engl J Med 1995; 28: 1726–31.

26. Davis SN, Shavers C, Costa F et al. Role of cortisol in the pathogenesis of deficient counterregulation after antecedent hypoglycemia in normal humans. J Clin Invest 1996; 98: 680–91.

27. Maran A, Lomas J, Macdonald IA et al. Lack of preservation of higher brain function during hypoglycaemia in patients with intensively-treated IDDM. Diabetologia 1995; 38: 1412–18.

28. Heller SR, Cryer PE. Reduced neuroendocrine and symptomatic responses to subsequent hypoglycemia after 1 episode of hypoglycemia in nondiabetic humans. Diabetes 1991; 40: 223–6.

29. Dagogo-Jack SE, Craft S, Cryer PE. Hypoglycemia-associated autonomic failure in insulin-dependent diabetes mellitus. J Clin Invest 1993; 91: 819–28.

30. Beer SF, Lawson C, Watkins PJ. Neurosis induced by home monitoring of blood glucose concentrations. Br Med J 1989; 298: 362.

31. Schade DS, Drumm DA, Eaton RP et al. Factitious brittle diabetes mellitus. Am J Med 1985; 78: 777–84.

32. Grunberger G, Weiner JL, Silverman R et al. Factitious hypoglycemia due to surreptitious administration of insulin. Diagnosis, treatment, and long-term follow-up. Ann Intern Med 1988; 108: 252–7.

33. Schuler G, Petersen KG, Khalaf AN et al. Insulin abuse in long-standing IDDM. Diabet Res Clin Pract 1989; 6: 145–8.

34. Hardy KJ, Burge MR, Boyle PJ et al. A treatable cause of recurrent severe hypoglycemia. Diabetes Care 1994; 17: 722–4.
35. ter Braak EW, Appelman AM, van de Laak M et al. Clinical characteristics of type 1 diabetic patients with and without severe hypoglycemia. Diabetes Care 2000; 23: 1467–71.
36. Farrell FJ, Keeffe EB. Diabetic gastroparesis. Dig Dis 1995; 13: 291–300.
37. Kimmerle R, Heinemann L, Delecki A et al. Severe hypoglycemia; incidence and predisposing factors in 85 pregnancies of Type 1 diabetic women. Diabet Care 1992; 15: 1034–7.
38. Linde J, Nilsson LH, Barany FR. Diabetes and hypoglycemia in chronic pancreatitis. Scand J Gastroenterol 1977; 12: 369–73.
39. Sjoberg RJ, Kidd GS. Pancreatic diabetes mellitus. Diabet Care 1989; 12: 715–24.
40. Avogaro A, Beltramello P, Gnudi L et al. Alcohol intake impairs glucose counterregulation during acute insulin-induced hypoglycemia in IDDM patients. Evidence for a critical role of free fatty acids. Diabetes 1993; 42: 1626–34.
41. Kerr D, Macdonald IA, Heller SR et al. Alcohol intoxication causes hypoglycaemia unawareness in healthy volunteers and patients with Type 1 (insulin-dependent) diabetes. Diabetologia 1990; 33: 216–21.
42. Luthra YK, Donaldson D. Lessons to be learned: a case study approach. Severe hypoglycaemia in insulin-dependent diabetes mellitus (IDDM) – living to tell the tale. J R Soc Health 1997; 117: 377–80.
43. Kitzmiller JL, Main E, Ward B et al. Insulin lispro and the development of proliferative diabetic retinopathy during pregnancy. Diabet Care 1999; 22: 874–6.
44. Buchbinder A, Miodovnik M, Khoury J et al. Is the use of insulin lispro safe in pregnancy? J Matern Fetal Neonatal Med 2002; 11: 232–7.
45. Fanelli CG, Epifano L, Rambotti AM et al. Meticulous prevention of hypoglycemia normalizes the glycemic thresholds of most of neuro-endocrine responses to, symptoms of, and cognitive function during hypoglycemia in intensively treated patients with short-term IDDM. Diabetes 1993; 42: 1683–9.
46. Cranston I, Lomas J, Maran A et al. Restoration of hypoglycaemia unawareness in patients with long-duration insulin-dependent diabetes. Lancet 1994; 344: 283–7.
47. Dagogo-Jack SE, Rattarasarn C, Cryer PE. Reversal of hypoglycemia unawareness, but not counterregulation, in IDDM. Diabetes 1994; 43: 1426–34.
48. Pickup JC, Keen H, Parsons JA et al. Continuous subcutaneous insulin infusion: an approach to achieving normoglycaemia. Br Med J 1978; 1: 204–7.
49. Locke DR, Rigg LA. Hypoglycemic coma associated with subcutaneous insulin infusion by portable pump. Diabet Care 1981; 4: 389–91.

50. Diabetes Control and Complications Trial Research Group. Implementation of treatment protocols in the Diabetes Control and Complications Trial. Diabet Care 1995; 18: 361–76.

51. Bode BW, Steed RD, Davidson PC. Reduction in severe hypoglycemia with long-term continuous subcutaneous insulin infusion in type I diabetes. Diabet Care 1996; 19: 324–7.

52. Pickup J, Keen H. Continuous subcutaneous insulin infusion at 25 years: evidence base for the expanding use of insulin pump therapy in type 1 diabetes. Diabet Care 2002; 25: 593–8.

53. Schade DS, Drum DA, Duckworth WC et al. The etiology of incapacitating brittle diabetes. Diabet Care 1985; 8: 12–20.

54. Berger M, Mühlhauser I. Implementation of intensified insulin therapy: a European perspective. Diabet Med 1995; 12: 201–8.

55. Muhlhauser I, Berger M. Diabetes education and insulin therapy: when will they ever learn? J Intern Med 1993; 233: 321–6.

56. Muhlhauser I, Jorgens V, Berger M et al. Bicentric evaluation of a teaching and treatment programme for type 1 (insulin-dependent) diabetic patients: improvement of metabolic control and other measures of diabetes care for up to 22 months. Diabetologia 1983; 25: 470–6.

57. Pieber TR, Brunner GA, Schnedl WJ et al. Evaluation of a structured outpatient group education program for intensive insulin therapy. Diabet Care 1995; 18: 625–30.

58. DAFNE Study Group. Training in flexible, intensive insulin management to enable dietary freedom in people with type 1 diabetes: dose adjustment for normal eating (DAFNE) randomised controlled trial. Br Med J 2002; 325: 746.

59. Bott S, Bott U, Berger M et al. Intensified insulin therapy and the risk of severe hypoglycaemia. Diabetologia 1997; 40: 926–32.

60. Muhlhauser I, Bruckner I, Berger M et al. Evaluation of an intensified insulin treatment and teaching programme as routine management of type 1 (insulin-dependent) diabetes. The Bucharest–Dusseldorf Study. Diabetologia 1987; 30: 681–90.

61. Cox DJ, Gonder-Frederick L, Polonsky W et al. Blood glucose awareness training (BGAT-2): long-term benefits. Diabet Care 2001; 24: 637–42.

62. Williams G, Pickup JC. The natural history of brittle diabetes. Diabet Res 1988; 7: 13–18.

chapter 8

Unstable diabetes in childhood and adolescence

Stephen Greene and Ray Newton

Any health carer advising on children and adolescents with type 1 diabetes is well aware of the instability of diabetes and that 'good' glycaemic control in this age range is often difficult to achieve, with adolescence a well-recognized period of overall poor glycaemic control. Along with this poor glycaemic control may come episodes of clinical instability – diabetic ketoacidosis (DKA) and/or hypoglycaemia – and the potential development of microvascular complications is brought into stark focus in this age group.

Glycaemic control in childhood and adolescence

Several surveys of large cohorts show conclusively an inexorable deterioration in glycaemic control from childhood through adolescence: Diabetes Control and Complications Trial (DCCT),[1] Danish Study Group,[2] French Study Group[3] and Scottish Study Group for the Care of the Young Diabetic (SSGCYD).[4] Our data in Scotland from the DIABAUD2 project showed the 11–15-year-old patients running an average HbA$_{1c}$ of 9.6% (girls) and 9.4% (boys) against in the younger age group (4 to 10 years of age), 8.7% (girls) and 8.7% (boys) (Figure 8.1). In both young children and teenagers there is a skewed distribution of glycated haemoglobin, with some children and teenagers having extremely poor metabolic control; in Scotland less than 25% of young people maintain their HbA$_{1c}$ under 8%.

The Hvidore Study Group on Childhood Diabetes examined blood glucose control in an international cross section of children and adolescents in 22 centres from 18 countries. Mean glycated haemoglobin for the cohort of 2873 children and adolescents was 8.6% (HbA$_{1c}$).[5] This was equivalent to 8.3% in the DCCT study and compared well to the intensive-treated group of teenagers in that study who had a mean HbA$_{1c}$ of 8.1%. Control deteriorated significantly throughout adolescence, despite an increase in insulin dose and the insulin regimen per se (2, 3, 4 or more injections of insulin per day) appeared to make no significant impact on this deterioration. Despite this apparent lack of effect of the insulin regimen, striking differences in the mean HbA$_{1c}$ control obtained in the centres occurred. Like our study in Scotland, no obvious factors determining glycaemic control emerged from this limited assessment of the patients' clinical management and the resources available to each centre.

Factors influencing poor glycaemic control

Physiological changes in glucose metabolism during adolescence

There appears to be increasing insulin 'resistance' in adolescence, reflected by changes in fasting insulin levels moving from childhood into puberty.[6] There are also major changes in the insulin-like growth factor 1 binding protein and growth hormone concentration in association with the puberty growth spurt.[7] We have recently shown marked 'insulin resistance' in normal teenagers in their response to a standard meal,[8] raising the concern over emerging type 2 diabetes phenotype in a large percentage of the young population. This, taken together

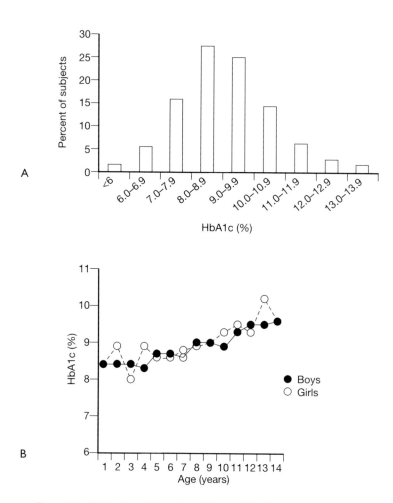

Figure 8.1 *Distribution of glycosylated haemoglobin (HbA₁c) in 1670 children and teenagers throughout Scotland. (A) Percentage achieving particular HbA₁c result. (B) Change with age, confirming deterioration in adolescence. (Data from DIABAUD2 Project by the Scottish Study Group for the Care of the Young Diabetic: n = 1670 patients; <15 years of age; reference 4.)*

with the emerging 'epidemic' of obesity in the young[9] and true clinical type 2 diabetes in adolescence,[10] is of concern to the type 1 population, where in theory the two insulin problems may coexist.

These physiological changes in glucose metabolism appear to be heightened in adolescents with type 1 diabetes. There appears to be an apparent need for an increase in insulin dosage to maintain a similar level of glycaemia moving from childhood to adolescence. Insulin-like growth factor 1 decreases significantly in the puberty years and there are major increases in IGF binding protein and growth hormone concentration.[7] Body composition changes can be quite marked in teenagers with diabetes, particularly in females.[11]

Behavioural, social and cultural changes in adolescence

Adolescents with diabetes are at a critical period. They are required to take responsibility for the management of their own diabetes,[12-14] and experience the relationship between their own actions, blood glucose levels and physical symptoms, which all influence their beliefs about diabetes and its management. These are formative years in the development of such beliefs, which, once fully integrated and accepted by the young person, may prove difficult to change. Therefore, they are in the unenviable position of facing the same developmental tasks and demands as all young people, but with the additional challenge of learning to manage their diabetes. The main challenge is to improve diabetes control through this transitional phase, without depriving young people of the appropriate age-related experiences.[15]

There is a wealth of literature on the psychological aspects of paediatric chronic illness, and diabetes in particular. Research has focused primarily on the relationship between adolescents and their families, with support and cohesion within the families consistently associated with better metabolic control and self-care.[16] Furthermore, early responsibility, accompanied by lack of parental involvement, for diabetes care is predictive of lower concordance, poor control and diabetic ketoacidosis.[17] However, there is a paucity of research on the role of the adolescent's peer group in relation to concordance, at a time when peer influence becomes important. Importantly it has been recommended that 'greater attention be paid to the social context' in which the adolescent lives.[18-20] The few studies that have been conducted indicate that peers are an important source of emotional support, and that this support is essential for optimal self-care and emotional well-being.[21–23]

Our group investigated the macro- and micro-cultural influences on the health strategies and beliefs of young people and professional health carers in adolescents with diabetes. In a cross-cultural study in Scotland and Italy, we used anthropological methodology that highlighted significant social and cultural influences on concordance with diabetes regimens.[24,25] In practical terms, the following occurred in the UK diabetes service:

- 'Good controllers' were more likely to be rewarded with less clinic visits, intensifying their sense of isolation.
- Responsibility was encouraged at an early age, separating them from family and peer support.
- Parents and peers were excluded at an age irrespective of development; i.e. categorization was by age, not by individual ability and preference.
- Exclusion of the parents obscured non-concordance, suggesting 'normal progress towards adulthood and independence'.
- Breaking down of reciprocal social networks providing community support of the young. This contrasted with considerable reciprocity between the health carers (e.g. conferences, team meetings, social support network).

Health care professionals comply with British social pressures to concentrate on the individuality of their patients, irrespective of their social situations, to make them accountable for their own illness. There is a mismatch between the health goals of the young person with diabetes and their health care professionals supporting them. This is compounded by the 'medicalization of adolescence': i.e. the expectation that adolescence is a medical entity and leads automatically to disruption of health. Health carers expect poor concordance in young people and there is a notion of low success and 'good concordance is viewed as abnormal in this age'. This leads to the expectation that the diabetes strategies are damned in this group from the outset.

Unmanageable diabetes in the young ('brittle diabetes')

The expectations after the introduction of insulin of a 'cure' for diabetes did not occur in all patients, and from the beginning it was commonly a difficult disease to manage, although, even in the young, good metabolic control was obtainable by rigid attention to detail: 4–6 injections per day (even of relatively impure insulin), meticulous attention to diet, obsessive monitoring of diabetes and regular sustained exercise. However, all patients did not achieve the desired outcome and medical practitioners began to suggest that 'bad control equalled bad patients', despite the inability of the diabetes management regimens to replicate the intricate homeostatic biochemical and physiological mechanisms that relate to insulin and glucose balance.

At the end of the spectrum of 'bad control' are a small number of patients, with not only high ambient blood glucose concentration but also with 'swinging' symptoms: frequent episodes of hypoglycaemia (often nocturnal) and hospital admissions for DKA. They became to be known as having brittle diabetes and were first described in textbooks on diabetes in the late 1920s and early 1930s. Subsequently, Tattersall defined the state as 'patients whose lives are constantly disrupted by episodes of hyperglycaemia or hypoglycaemia, whatever the cause'. [26]

From their early descriptions physicians tried to elucidate brittle diabetes in terms of intrinsic problems with the diabetes (abnormal counter-regulatory hormone reaction, pituitary abnormalities, coexisting diseases associated with diabetes) or abnormal reaction to the insulin injection (abnormal insulin absorption, insulin degradation products, high insulin antibody production). With the introduction of home blood glucose monitoring, newer insulin preparations, continuous subcutaneous insulin infusion (CSII) and automatic pancreas machines such as the Biostator, the 1970s and 1980s saw a series of investigations in the UK and the USA into brittle diabetes, attempting to unearth the responsible organic defect.[27,28] Interestingly all of the groups began to describe a relatively homogeneous collection of patients who were being referred for investigation of extreme brittleness. These were nearly all young women ranging in age from late childhood into their early twenties. They were C-peptide negative, had poor glycaemic control, were often prescribed high doses of insulin and yet many were significantly overweight. Detailed studies of these patients, particularly by the Newcastle[29] and Guy's Hospital group,[30] and by Schade's group in the USA,[31] revealed a high incidence of marked behavioural abnormalities (factitious disease, malingering, communication disorders). The Guy's group, after many years of searching for organic causes of brittle diabetes, firmly stated that: 'the most likely cause of rapidly developing hyperglycaemia and ketosis in these patients remains insulin deficiency due to the patient interrupting insulin administration'.[24]

The patients described above were often referred to the investigating units for detailed study after several years of major difficulties in their home base. For any centre that cares for young people with type 1 diabetes for several years, it is likely that there is always a current case that the medical teams struggle to support. However, as the understanding of brittle diabetes has emerged over the years, we believe a wider interpretation should now be in place. Tattersall's definition suggested constant disruption. We believe that many patients fall into a broader description of brittleness, underpinned by therapeutic insulin deficiency, with occasional (even just one) life-threatening episodes of DKA and/or nocturnal hypoglycaemia, who have periods of relative stability, although usually poor glycaemic control. These teenagers may have overt behavioural problems and/or difficult home, school or relationship circumstances.[32] With this wider description many will recognize such patients in their clinic, giving the teenager a 'bad name'.

Specific reasons for instability

Insulin omission
Insulin deficiency, producing erratic control and, subsequently, brittle diabetes with episodes of DKA, is most likely due to insulin omission.

Manipulation and factitious insulin delivery have been seen in the most severe psychologically disturbed patients. Several case reports have been published of hidden insulin, diluted insulin preparations and tampering with intravenous and intraperitoneal catheters.[33] Most of these have come to light following extensive hospital investigation.

More recently, insulin omission has emerged as the common phenomenon to account for the vast majority of episodes of DKA in the older teenager known to have diabetes. Although clinicians had suspected it since the initial treatment of diabetes, direct evidence has only recently been forthcoming. Capillary blood glucose testing and glycated haemoglobin estimation in the 1980s firmly established the suboptimal control of many young people with diabetes. It was appreciated that a lack of concordance with the prescribed therapy regimens (insulin and diet) may be the basis for such poor control and agreed with the developing literature on the psychological impact of this chronic disease. As Steel so eloquently stated: 'there is a reluctance to believe that patients would deliberately cheat their doctor and, after all "she is such a nice girl she would never do anything like that".'[34]

In our unit, Thompson et al described the differences between young people with DKA and older more established diabetes.[35] No specific cause was established in the majority and they responded dramatically to simple fluid and insulin therapy. The often-quoted reason of infection as the cause of the DKA was not established. More specifically we were able to show that the reason for DKA in young people was insulin omission. The DARTS/MEMO programme allows for a direct measure of insulin prescription in the Tayside region. Using the community health index number (CHI), a six-figure unique identifier, we are able to measure individual encashment of prescriptions. We examined in 90 young people with type 1 diabetes (aged under 25 years) the insulin prescription rate over 1 year and compared the encashment rate with the prescribed insulin dose through the clinics.[36] In the older teenager we found a failure to collect all of their prescribed insulin over 1 year in over 50%, with on average 28% collecting less than one third of their insulin. A low

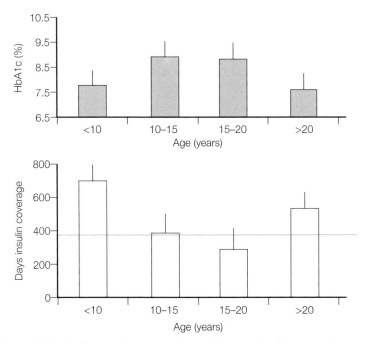

Figure 8.2 *Lack of concordance in insulin encashment and influence on glycaemic control. Insulin omission in the middle teenage years is associated with poor glycated haemoglobin levels. Data from DARTS / MEMO.*[38]

encashment of insulin was associated with a high admission rate for DKA and overall poor control (Figure 8.2).

In the DIABUAD2 study daily insulin dose (units/body weight/day) increased with age. There was a considerable spread in dose, with a significant proportion of patients prescribed >1.0 unit/kg/day. However, HbA_{1c} remained constant (and disappointingly poor) in this age group. One interpretation is that more insulin is required to overcome the insulin resistance of adolescence, just to stand still. Another explanation is that increasing insulin continues to be prescribed by health workers in ever-increasing doses, not realizing that teenagers are not taking a significant percentage of their insulin dose. We favour the latter explanation.

These data suggest to us that persisting poor control (HbA_{1c} >11.0%) in our clinic is usually synonymous with insulin deficiency secondary to a lack of concordance with prescribed insulin therapy.

Insulin, weight and eating disorders

Diabetes, particularly for girls, is a battleground for the powerful effect that insulin has on fat metabolism and the culturally unacceptable body images of excessive weight in modern society. 'High doses' of insulin are frequently used to achieve as low a blood glucose level as possible. The effect on the glucose levels may be for many at the expense of extra carbohydrate intake and alteration in body fat distribution and mass. Data from the Hvidore International Study Group confirms the 'excessive weight' of older teenage girls and we all have a group in our clinic with marked weight gain. For these girls this is their major problem.

The ability to translate the advice from the diabetes health professional into their home care management is not for the vast majority a lack of knowledge. Many studies have now revealed that the understanding of diabetes information in children, teenagers and their parents is high. It is the desire and the want to take this information forward that is the key to concordance with the diabetes regimens.[37] Therefore, it is not surprising that many teenagers 'learn' that insulin omission may be a ploy to be used in an attempt to keep weight down.

At the same time it has been accepted that there is a relatively higher incidence of eating disorders (anorexia nervosa, bulimia, binge eating) in, particularly, girls with diabetes.[38] With the realization that eating disorders are common in young people, it is not surprising that this is increased in diabetes, with its emphasis on diet as a treatment modality. The combination of insulin omission and erratic eating habits is a powerful tool to reduce weight or keep weight steady at the expense of poor glycaemic control. For many this is acceptable, even with the ensuing poor control and the risk of an episode of DKA.

Other diseases

Undoubtedly, a sudden change in the stability of the diabetes requires attention. Specific diseases are associated with diabetes and these may lead to erratic and brittle control. In the young other autoimmune diseases are the most likely. Thyroid antibodies have been reported in 10 to even 50% of diabetic patients under the age of 25 years.[39]

Hypothryoidism or thryrotoxicosis, however, are rarer (<5–10%), but nevertheless should be considered in any case of deteriorating control – similarly, asymptomatic coeliac and Addison's disease. Chronic infection (e.g. tuberculosis) is now no longer increased in diabetes. However, all children with diabetes are open to other general childhood illnesses that should be considered (infection, anaemia, leukaemia, etc.).

Complications and the teenager with diabetes

The DCCT, along with several other clinical studies, confirmed the association between long-term suboptimal blood glucose control and the risk of microvascular complications. Persistent poor control in teenagers increases that risk considerably with a concern for the development of 'malignant' microvascular change, particularly retinopathy. Perhaps, not surprisingly, long-term diabetic complications are considerably higher in adults with diabetes who have had a period of poor control in their teenage years. It is likely that the complication risk in stable patients is falling, whereas they are increasing in the erratic and poorly controlled cases. They also have a poorer quality of life and more complications in pregnancy. Tragically, many will also die young from the severe episodes of hypoglycaemia and DKA. Certain complications of diabetes may well contribute to instability of glycaemic control.

Gastric stasis, as a form of autonomic neuropathy, has been reported, and it is suggested to be commoner than appreciated.[40] It is likely, however, that this complication of poor glycaemic control is a secondary and reversible phenomena rather than the primary cause of the brittleness of the diabetes itself. Improving control reverses the symptoms of bloatedness, abdominal pains and vomiting.

Frequent episodes of hypoglycaemia are part of the poor control seen in the teenage years. Hypoglycaemia alone with stable acceptable glycaemic control (HbA_{1c} <8.5%) is seen frequently in children and young people. The hypoglycaemia is usually reactive to exercise or omission of food (especially in the young child) or during periods of illness. Severe episodes of hypoglycaemia, in association with poor glycemic control and episodes of DKA, are the picture of unstable adolescence in diabetes. A separate factor to be considered in teenagers is alcohol use. This affects girls as frequently as boys these days, and is particularly associated with severe nocturnal hypoglycaemia. There is some evidence to suggest that a significant proportion of the 'dead in bed' syndrome described in young people with diabetes is alcohol related.

Care strategies for the adolescent

The approach to poor glycaemic control in the adolescent with diabetes has to be made on two levels: the individual patient with erratic control and life-threatening episodes of hypoglycaemia and DKA; the general approach to the delivery of the service for diabetes in an attempt to minimize the problem. At the root of both, we believe, is the aim of improving adherence with the diabetes regimens.

Diabetes therapy

As always, specific therapy should be tailored to the individual patient. Insulin, diet and exercise still remain the cornerstones of therapy, as for all age groups, with advice not to smoke and limit alcohol consumption. Pre-pregnancy advice about diabetes is essential.

These strategies have to be tailored to the individual's rapidly changing lifestyle, education programme and social situation. In the modern vernacular 'wicked man; dead easy, eh!' Can the above be achieved or are they 'in our dreams!'. Yes, for some teenagers aggressive treatment of their diabetes with multiple injections or insulin pumps, close control of carbohydrate intake and regular exercise is the preferred and desired option. Teenagers, like all people with diabetes, must be given the options and helped to make decisions with which they are comfortable. Although there is limited evidence on the effectiveness of insulin regimens other than conventional twice daily, our experience of more intensive regimens suggests that they are acceptable and have good results in some teenagers. This is provided individuals are willing to adhere to the necessary injection and monitoring regimen. Our approach is to offer and try, but be willing to change frequently.

Behavioural and social therapy

No specific insulin regimen, however, can be prescribed in isolation of a behavioural and social package: a social support network. The overt severely brittle patient requires detailed psychological and often psychiatric support and therapy. While there are often severe social and family problems, the patient's presentation (malingering, factitious therapy, interference) suggests a specific psychiatric problem: personality disorder, depression, schizophrenia, anorexia nervosa and bulimia. In the younger child with unstable diabetes and unusual occurrences, consideration should be given to a psychiatric disorder in the parent, i.e. Munchausen syndrome by proxy.

These overtly unstable patients with chronic imminently life-threatening very poor glycaemic control usually present over a considerable time and may reach a point where the diabetes team request 'outside' professional help. Perhaps a failing of our services is the reluctance to consider these approaches sooner. The desire to continue to investigate these cases for an organic cause, the manipulation and fabrication of the patients and the lack of psychiatric resources usually results in a significant delay in the effective psychiatric treatment being instigated.

For the less florid patient with erratic symptoms and poor control, most patients can and should be supported within the diabetes clinic and by the diabetes team. These patients do not have overt psychiatric disorders. They are usually reacting to difficult periods in their life, which have a basis either in social problems (e.g. parents divorce, alcoholism and drugs, unemployment, poor education) or emotional difficulties (e.g. relationship difficulties, school or work problems, general low esteem and difficulties in accepting and coping with the diabetes). Specific diabetes problems sometimes add to the difficulties: e.g. needle phobia, overweight, fear of complications, fear of hypoglycaemia.

Although insulin omission is the basic problem, stark confrontation is problematic and has to be handled with care and compassion. Many young people in our experience accept explanation about our understanding that insulin omission occurs very frequently, with no judgement attached. Even if they deny omitting their insulin, working with the patient must continue. Support and frequent contact often encourages returning back to the routine of diabetes. Lapses should not be viewed with despair. Having diabetes is a marathon, not a sprint. Many of the professionals move on and out of the patient's life. Many young people reject an aggressive, dictatorial approach. Constant encouragement, regular factual information and consistency of the messages are important. The patients should be seen frequently by the team members (physicians, dietitians and nurses) in a variety of environments. Consideration should be given to a multiple injection regimen (e.g. pre-meal fast-acting insulin with a long-acting preparation before supper). This is, however, not a quick fix. For many it will be inappropriate and a simple daily regimen of two injections a day is a better option. It may be appropriate to go for suboptimal control (i.e. HbA_{1c} running around 10%) but with no episodes of DKA or hypoglycaemia for a short period. Given the continuum of association of poor glycaemic control with the risk of complications, rather than a threshold effect, this may be an acceptable trade-off.

For many the discussions will be detailed and frequent. It may be necessary to include other family members. While respecting the independence of the teenager and the parents, we do not automatically exclude either just because a certain age has been reached. Open and honest discussion is in our opinion more successful in the long run.

The general lack of adherence with the therapy regimens is a challenge for all involved in the care of young people with type 1 diabetes. Our own observations using methodology from social science has led us to the view that in an individualistic society, such as the UK, the empowerment given to young people and acknowledged by adults, 'allows them' to reject the rigours of the diabetes regimens. In a more egalitarian society, where a collective approach to support and direction is given, teenagers seem to accept the diabetes routine more as a matter of course. Novel strategies of care in the UK are required to overcome these difficulties in concording with the diabetes regimens and care plans.

For instance, the DCCT suggested strongly that the change to a more intensive insulin regimen (four or more daily insulin injections or pump insulin therapy) was the reason for producing 'good' glycaemic control. However, following the publication of the trial a debate ensued, suggesting that the 'clinical support package' (intensive medical follow-up; additional nursing and dietetic input; frequent contact) was the main factor in the improvement of control. The Hvidore Study demonstrated that there are centre differences in glycaemic control, particularly in teenagers. Further analysis of the data suggests that differences in the mean metabolic control of various centres operated early in the course of the disease. This suggests that the 'intensive therapy package' for the management of the diabetes is set in place from the beginning of the management of the diabetic child and teenager. Given that adjustment for significant associations with glycaemic control did not explain the centre differences, there appears to be factors not analysed in the DIABAUD2 survey (e.g. deployment of resources, organization of the clinical structure, strategies of care, clinic philosophy) that appear to influence glycaemic control in individuals. These must operate differently in different centres. From discussion within the SSGCYD, the 'best' centre has a policy of frequent contact (both medical and nursing), with at least monthly formal advice (more if required), together with a rapid 'troubleshooting' service, frequent change in insulin regimen, with no fixed 'favourite' and the aim of a near normal target for HbA_{1c} (<7.5%). We speculate that utilization of optimum resources is the key factor to achieving good glycaemic control.

Social outings, camps, etc.
As part of the development of a social support network, discussions and specific advice about diabetes will need to be delivered outside the clinical setting. Observational evidence has highlighted the impact

that peer pressure can have in a surrounding conducive to sharing the difficulties about diabetes in a young person. Several years of contact with young people through the Youth Diabetes Project (Firbush Summer Camp and the Youth Diabetes Meeting)[41] has acknowledged the concerns of young people with diabetes and, for many, these activities have been the only social support that they have experienced about diabetes.

New possibilities exist through new forms of communication. 'Cyber space' has the potential for social support to be delivered to a large number of patients, with not only information about diabetes reaching teenagers but also support in the form of directives, reminders, challenges, etc. It is hoped that the world of the adolescent with diabetes does genuinely become a smaller, and therefore a more comfortable, place in the very near future.

In summary, to combat the instability of diabetes in this age group, we present a view that adolescents with type 1 diabetes should be approached with an individualized diabetes management plan, leaning towards an intensive insulin regimen with available psychological and psychiatric assessment and treatment if required. For individual patients, support, compassion and detailed attention is required over a lengthy period. Novel care approaches need to be considered to encourage more teenagers in the UK to treat their diabetes aggressively, and these should incorporate social structures necessary for concordance with the diabetes management strategies.

References

1. The Diabetes Control and Complications Trial Research Group. The effect of intensive treatment of diabetes on the development and progression of long term complications in insulin dependent diabetes mellitus. N Engl J Med 1993; 329: 977–86.
2. Mortensen HB, Marinelli K, Norgaard K et al and the Danish Study Group of Diabetes in Childhood. A nationwide cross-sectional study of urinary albumin excretion rate, arterial blood pressure and blood glucose control in Danish children with Type 1 diabetes mellitus. Diabet Med 1990; 7: 887–97.

3. Rosilio M, Cotton JB, Wieliczko MC et al. Factors associated with glycaemic control. A cross-sectional nationwide study in 2,579 French children with Type 1 diabetes. The French Pediatric Diabetes Group. Diabetes Care 1998; 21: 1146–53.

4. Greene SA on behalf of the Scottish Study Group for the Care of the Young Diabetic. Factors influencing glycaemic control in young people with type 1 diabetes in Scotland: A population based study (Diabaud2). Diabet Med 1999; 16(suppl. 1); 9.

5. Mortensen HB, Hougaard P. Comparison of metabolic control in a cross sectional study of 2873 children and adolescents with IDDM from 18 countries. The Hvidore Study Group on Childhood Diabetes. Diabetes Care 1997; 20: 714–20.

6. Hindmarsh PC, Matthews DR, Silvio LDI et al. Relation between height velocity and fasting insulin concentrations. Arch Dis Child 1988; 63: 665–6.

7. Dunger DB, Cheetham TD, Holly JMP, Matthews DR. Does recombinant insulin like growth factor (IGFI) have a role in the treatment of insulin-dependent diabetes mellitus during adolescence? Acta Paediatr Suppl 1993; 388: 49–52.

8. Green F, Khan F, Kennedy G et al. Syndrome X and endothelial function in children. Diabet Med 1999; 16(suppl 1): 5.

9. White E, Wilson AC, Greene SA et al. Body mass index centile charts to assess fatness of British children. Arch Dis Child 1995; 72: 38–41.

10. Pinhas-Hamiel O, Zeitler P. Type 2 diabetes in adolescents, no longer rare. Pediatr Rev 1998; 19: 434–5.

11. Gregory JW, Wilson AC, Greene SA. Obesity among adolescents with diabetes. Diabet Med 1992; 9: 344–7.

12. Allen DA, Tennen H, McGrade BJ et al. Parent and child perceptions of the management of juvenile diabetes. J Pediatr Psychol 1983; 8: 129–41.

13. Burroughs T, Harris MA, Pontious SL, Santiago JV. Research on social support in adolescents with IDDM. Diabet Educ 1997; 23: 438–48.

14. Drotar D. Relating parent and family functioning to the psychological adjustment of children with chronic health conditions. J Pediatr Psychol 1997; 22: 149–66.

15. Hauser, ST, Jacobson AM, Lavori P et al. Adherence among children and adolescents with insulin-dependent diabetes mellitus over a four-year longitudinal follow-up. J Pediatr Psychol 1990; 15: 527–42.

16. Anderson, BJ, Auslander WF, Jung KC et al. Assessing family sharing of diabetes responsibilities. J Pediatr Psychol 1990; 15: 477–92.

17. Anderson, B, Ho J, Brackett J et al. Parental involvement in diabetes management tasks. J Pediatr 1997; 130: 257–65.

18. White K, Kolman ML, Wexler P et al. Unstable diabetes and unstable families. Pediatrics 1984; 73: 749–55.

19. Montemayor R. The study of personal relationships during adolescence.

In: Personal relationships during adolescence. Sage, London, 1994, pp 1–6.

20. Glasgow RE, Anderson BJ. Future directions for research on pediatric chronic disease management: lessons from diabetes. J Pediatr Psychol 1995; 20: 389–402.

21. La Greca AM. Peer influences in pediatric chronic illness: an update. J Pediatr Psychol 1992; 17: 775–84.

22. La Greca AM, Auslander WF, Greco P et al. I get by with a little help from my family and friends: adolescents' support for diabetes care. J Pediatr Psychol 1995; 20: 449–76.

23. Skinner TC, Hampson SE. Social support and personal models of diabetes in relation to self-care and well-being in adolescents with type 1 diabetes mellitus. J Adolesc 1998; 21: 703–15.

24. Greene AC. Health carers' and young peoples' conceptualisations of chronic illness: an anthropological interpretation of diabetes mellitus. PhD thesis, University St Andrews, Scotland, UK, 2000.

25. Greene AC, Tripaldi M, McKeirnan P et al. Promoting empowerment in young people with type 1 diabetes. Diabet Med 1999; 16: 20.

26. Tattersall RB. Brittle diabetes re-visited: the Third Arnold Bloom Memorial Lecture. Diabet Med 1997; 14: 99–110.

27. Williams G, Pickup JC, Keen H. Continuous intravenous insulin infusion in the management of brittle diabetes: etiologic and therapeutic implications. Diabetes Care 1985; 8: 21–7.

28. Schade DS, Duckworth WC. In search of the subcutaneous insulin resistance syndrome. N Engl J Med 1986; 315: 143–47.

29. Gill GV, Alberti KGMM. Outcome of brittle diabetes. Br Med J 1991; 303: 285–6.

30. Williams G, Pickup JC. The natural history of brittle diabetes. Diabet Res 1988; 7: 13–18.

31. Schade DS. Brittle diabetes: strategies, diagnosis and treatment. Diabet Metab Rev 1988; 4: 371–90.

32. Williams G, Gill G, Pickup JC. Brittle diabetes. Br Med J 1991; 303: 714.

33. Gill GV. The spectrum of brittle diabetes. J Roy Soc Med 1992; 85: 259–61.

34. Steel JM. 'Such a nice girl'. Lancet 1994; 344: 765–6.

35. Thompson CJ, Cummings F, Chalmers J, Newton RW. Abnormal insulin treatment behaviour: a major cause of ketoacidosis in the young adult. Diabet Med 1995; 12: 429–32.

36. Morris AM, Boyle DIR, McMahon AD et al for the DARTS/MEMO collaboration. Adherence to insulin treatment, glycaemic control and keto-acidosis in IDDM. Lancet 1997; 350: 1505–10.

37. Howells L, Wilson AC, Skinner TC et al. A randomised controlled trial of the effect of negotiated telephone support on glycaemic control in young people with type 1 diabetes. Diabet Med 2002; 19: 643–8.

38. Steel JM, Young RJ, Lloyd GG, MacIntyre CCA. Abnormal eating attitudes in young insulin-dependent diabetics. Br J Psychiatry 1989; 1555: 515–21.
39. Neufeld M, Maclaren NK, Riley WJ et al. Islet cell and other organ specific antibodies in US Caucasians and Blacks with insulin dependent diabetes mellitus. Diabetes 1980; 8: 589–92.
40. Campbell IW, Heading RC, Tothill P et al. Gastric emptying in diabetic autonomic neuropathy. Horm Metab Res Suppl 1980; 9: 81–6.
41. Davies RR, Newton RW. Progress in the Youth Diabetes Project. Pract Diabet 1989; 6: 6.

chapter 9

Brittle diabetes in the elderly

Sue Benbow and Michael Gallagher

Introduction

Europe, and the rest of the western world, represents an ageing society. In England, for example, the number of people over 65 has more than doubled since the 1930s and there are now more people aged over 60 than under 16. Approximately 7% of the population is aged 75 or more and the number of people aged over 85 has increased more than 5.5 fold since 1951.[1]

Diabetes is already common in elderly UK citizens and numbers will increase as the population ages. The prevalence of diabetes is approximately 10% in the UK elderly[2] and even higher in those of Asian origin.[3] There also appears to be an increasing prevalence of diabetes in the elderly population,[4] partly attributable to improved detection but also due to a true increase in prevalence.[5] Although the majority of these patients will have type 2 diabetes, type 1 diabetes exists in the elderly due to survival into old age but, in addition, can uncommonly occur de novo in this population.[6,7] A Danish study showed that the annual incidence of type 1 diabetes is constant at 8.2/100 000 per year from the fourth to ninth decades.[8]

Elderly patients with diabetes are more likely to have other co-morbid conditions, cognitive impairment and depression than matched controls.[9] Compared with younger subjects the elderly are also more likely to be dependent, socially isolated and taking multiple medications.

Therefore, on a background of increasing traditionally associated macrovascular and microvascular complications, the elderly person with diabetes potentially has to deal with the effects of cognitive disorders, depression and falls as well as other geriatric conditions. It is therefore surprising that the older person with diabetes has been historically relatively neglected[10] and continues to be so.[11]

Poorly controlled diabetes with glycaemic instability exists in all ages, but 'brittleness' has classically been thought to be a problem of the young. This chapter will examine what evidence there is that brittle diabetes exists in the elderly population, review the characteristics and possible aetiological factors, and finally discuss the options for investigation and management in this age group.

Does brittle diabetes exist in the elderly?

The various definitions of brittleness have been discussed elsewhere,[12] but in the elderly population there are few reports on the subject of brittle diabetes no matter what definition is used.

It had been noted in a study of episodes of uncontrolled diabetes (plasma glucose over 33 mmol/l and venous bicarbonate less than 14 mmol/l), that a third of episodes were in patients over the age of 50.[13] However this study did not involve repeated episodes of hyperglycaemia and therefore is not a 'brittle' study, although it is sometimes quoted as such.

Another study examined recurrent ketoacidosis, in patients aged more than 12, over a 15-year period.[14] Recurrent ketoacidosis was defined as 3 or more episodes in a 4–year period. Of 39 patients, 12 were under 20 years old, whereas 10 were 60 or older. A further paper described a sample of 6 elderly patients, where episodes of hypo- and hyperglycaemia led to lifestyle disruption.[15] Subsequently, a study of the prevalence of brittle diabetes in the UK identified a small but distinct group of older patients, in addition to the expected peak of brittle young females.[16] In this study brittleness was defined as 'insulin-dependent diabetes with glycaemic instability of any type leading to life disruption and/or prolonged hospitalizations'. More recently a further attempt has been made to define the characteristics of an elderly cohort, with a paper describing 55 patients with brittle diabetes aged 60 or over from across the UK,[17] using the definition described above.[16]

These studies confirm that brittle diabetes does exist in the over-sixties. However, there is insufficient data to give a true indication of its prevalence. The only study that has attempted this, in all ages, reported an overall prevalence of nearly 1 per 1000 adult diabetic patients,[16] with 17 patients aged 60–70, out of an adult brittle population of 323 (5%). Although Benbow et al[17] reported the largest group of elderly brittle patients so far, this was not designed as a prevalence study.

Age and sex distribution

In the early case series of elderly brittle diabetes,[15] 6 patients were described, with 5 being female. One patient was in their eighties. In the study by Benbow et al,[17] 71% were female. Patients ranged in age from 60 to 89 years old, with the majority in their eighth decade. Ninety per cent (90%) of elderly patients in a further study were also female.[14]

This female predominance would appear to concur with the excess of females reported elsewhere.[16,18] However, the apparent female excess in the elderly brittle population must obviously be approached with the caveat that there is existing female excess in the elderly.

Types of glycaemic instability

Existing data on brittle diabetes in younger patients have suggested that the majority of episodes are due to recurrent ketoacidosis.[16,18] For instance, Gill et al[16] found that recurrent ketoacidosis accounted for 59% of cases (Fig. 9.1A). This contrasts with the survey in the elderly,

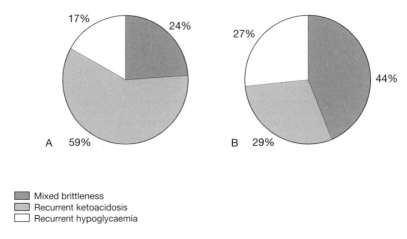

Mixed brittleness
Recurrent ketoacidosis
Recurrent hypoglycaemia

Figure 9.1 *Proportions of patients with the three major metabolic syndromes of brittleness according to age: (A) all ages (Gill et al[16]); (B) elderly (Benbow et al[17]).*

where brittleness was classed as mixed glycaemic instability in 44% followed by recurrent ketoacidosis in 29% and recurrent hypoglycaemia in 27%[17] (Fig. 9.1B). Griffith and Yudkin[15] similarly reported that all 6 of their patients were affected by both hyper- and hypoglycaemia. The information available to date would therefore seem to suggest a different pattern of brittleness between the younger and older age groups.

Aetiology

Although there have been a variety of theories on the causation of brittle diabetes, in the typical young patient it is now often thought to be self-induced and closely related to psychosocial problems.[12,19] Again, this contrasts with experience in the elderly group.

Chapman and colleagues[14] reported that all of the elderly patients had concurrent chronic illness, both medical and psychiatric, in contrast with the younger group. In 3 of the 6 patients in another small study, cognitive impairment was subsequently discovered and may have been a contributory factor to the glycaemic instability, although there was no obvious reason in any of the patients.[15] In one of the individuals, instability continued despite inpatient management of diabetes. Furthermore, a case report of an elderly patient with recurrent glycaemic instability (despite intensive self-management strategies and multiple-injection therapy) demonstrates the difficulties of finding an underlying cause for the problem.[20]

In a recent survey,[17] the diabetes team responsible for the patient's care felt the causes of brittleness to be multiple in two-thirds of cases. Single causes proposed included medical diseases in 14% and hypoglycaemic unawareness in 6%. In only 4 patients (8%) were cognitive-behavioural problems thought to be a predominant feature, although they probably contributed to the pathogenesis in a further 20%. No obvious cause was found in 3 patients. Unlike the younger brittle patients, in only 4 of the individuals was there any suggestion of deliberate manipulation of diabetes. However, in all 4 of these patients, there were also chronic non-diabetic medical conditions. It therefore appears that the underlying causes of brittleness contrast with that of the younger patients described elsewhere.

Social isolation may potentially contribute to brittleness[14] but elderly brittle patients live in a variety of social situations including residential accommodation.[17] However, in the latter study,[17] previous place of residence was not available and it is feasible that glycaemic instability contributed to the reason for people moving into the institution.[21]

Outcome

The mortality of acute diabetic complications, particularly hyperglycaemia, increases with age.[13,22] However, the outcome of true brittle diabetes in the elderly is unknown and such studies would obviously be relatively difficult to perform.

Specific problems in the elderly

Elderly patients with brittle diabetes present at least as difficult a challenge as the younger person, although the potential aetiological factors encompass a wider spectrum of disorders and conditions. Importantly, multiple precipitants may be involved and require careful investigation with corroborating evidence from a variety of sources. Similar issues can be involved in the elderly person with poorly controlled diabetes even if any of the definitions of 'brittleness' are not reached.

As discussed elsewhere,[12] the relationship between psychological stresses and young people with brittle diabetes usually dominates the clinical picture even if not initially obvious. This does not seem to be the major causal relationship in the elderly, although it is of course possible.[17] The following areas need to be reviewed in an attempt to clarify the situation and alleviate the problem in the elderly patient (Table 9.1).

Table 9.1 Factors in the elderly that potentially contribute to glycaemic instability

Insulin therapy and administration
Impaired recognition of poor control: e.g. reduced awareness of hypoglycaemia
Co-morbidity: e.g. multiple pathology, atypical presentation
Disability: e.g. arthritis, visual disease
Communication problems: e.g. deafness, dysphasia
Polypharmacy
Nutrition
Cognitive impairment
Depression
Social circumstances

Diabetes management and mismanagement

It is imperative not to assume that insulin administration is correct in the aged, as in the younger person. Although insulin prescription should be relatively straightforward, the potential for a variety of mistakes is increased in the aged. For instance, a comparison of insulin prescribed with that taken (type, timing, dosage, etc.) is necessary, along with a thorough review of the technique of injecting. Insulin devices can be difficult to use for some people and, even if previously adept, changing physical or cognitive function can cause difficulties. Elderly type 1 patients may still be mixing their own insulin, thereby increasing the possibility of dosage errors. If a partner or other carer is giving the insulin, then they similarly should be assessed.

The professional should review insulin dosage in the light of any change in circumstances, such as weight loss. Likewise, the ability to monitor blood glucose levels may become problematic with changes in vision, dexterity or cognitive function. Re-education may be necessary or, alternatively, education of carers (professional or otherwise) provided.

Recognition of poor control

Hyperglycaemia may be difficult to recognize for patient and doctor alike, with symptoms of thirst less prominent, acidotic breathing mistaken for heart failure or chest infection, and urinary frequency mistaken for infection or prostatism.

Likewise, hypoglycaemia in the elderly can differ from that in the younger person in a variety of ways, a subject that has recently been reviewed.[23] Some of these differences may be of practical importance in the aged person with hypoglycaemia, although only some can be influenced.

Blunted hormonal autonomic responses to hypoglycaemia have sometimes been reported[24] and there may be a reduction in symptom intensity in the elderly.[25] The symptoms of hypoglycaemia can also vary according to age.[23,26] The presence of neurological symptoms, for example, may be mistaken for cognitive impairment, cerebrovascular disease, or confusion (by professional or patient alike) rather than hypoglycaemia. Elderly patients may also have little knowledge of hypoglycaemia.[27]

Furthermore, the blood glucose threshold for generating symptoms may be lowered in the elderly[28] and, therefore by the time the individual suspects hypoglycaemia, they may not be able to act appropriately.[23]

Many type 1 patients are hypoglycaemic unaware: this is associated with duration of diabetes and leads to an increased risk of severe hypoglycaemia.[29] It is therefore not surprising that some elderly brittle patients were reported to be hypoglycaemic unaware.[17] Hypoglycaemia in the aged can have wider consequences than in the younger patient with physical trauma more likely.

Medical disease

As in the younger person, organic causes for brittleness need to be considered and excluded where possible. This may be more complex, as the elderly may present atypically. There are often multiple pathologies, and infection or malignancy may be occult. In addition to the recognized microvascular and macrovascular complications of diabetes, with concomitant increased morbidity and increased resource usage,[9,21,30,31] there are also more unappreciated complications. These include the cognitive problems discussed below, as well as physical disability, falls and fractures. Co-morbidity is more common with increasing age, even in those without diabetes.

Endocrine disease must be considered, as the symptomatology may be vague and non-specific. Addison's disease, causing hypoglycaemia, should be considered, as in the young. Hypopituitarism may likewise be difficult to recognize in the elderly person.[32]

Coeliac disease can present de novo in the elderly.[33] Recurrent urinary tract infections may present as incontinence rather than with symptoms of dysuria or frequency, and be exacerbated by hyperglycaemia.

Alcohol misuse is not the preserve of the young and should be considered as a potential cause of hypoglycaemia. However, medical causes are seldom the single major cause of problems with control in elderly brittle patients, and are more often a contributory factor.[17]

Disability

Common physical problems which may impinge on the ability to manage diabetes include stroke disease, arthritis affecting the hands and visual impairment. Poor vision may occur in the elderly for several reasons (not just diabetes-related): e.g. age-related macular degeneration and open-angle glaucoma. Other co-morbidities include significant cardiac or peripheral vascular disease, amputations or respiratory problems, all of which may further limit function. Elderly people with diabetes have been shown to have excess disability compared with a non-diabetic population even when diabetes complications are taken into account.[9,34,35]

Communication problems, such as deafness and dysphasia, may make the elucidation of brittleness more difficult than in the younger person.

Disabilities may not only cause difficulties with insulin administration and monitoring but may also hinder daily activities such as meal preparation and shopping and potentially limit access to care.

Drug effects and polypharmacy

Older patients are more likely to be prescribed and take multiple medications, some of which may interfere with diabetes control, e.g. steroids. The complexity of polypharmacy may also have implications for compliance, and can cause potential side effects such as renal impairment or anorexia. Drugs taken must be carefully ascertained as 'over-the-counter' prescriptions increase in availability, along with the usage of homeopathic remedies and medication borrowed from spouses or friends!

Nutrition

Formal dietary assessment should be performed, particularly when hypoglycaemia predominates. Undernutrition is well recognized as an area of concern in older people in general.[36,37] Nutritional deficiencies can be secondary to anorexia (itself due to disease or drugs), dysphagia following stroke or other neurological disease, depression or dementia. Social isolation or poverty, impaired mobility and difficulty in food preparation or access in the absence of sufficient support may compound these disorders. Even if meals are provided by 'meals on wheels' or other agencies, they may not be eaten for a myriad of reasons. Practical physical problems such as poor or absent dentition will make matters worse. There is no guarantee of adequate nutrition even when living in institutions.[38]

Monitoring of weight is important in the elderly, particularly when hypoglycaemia and loss of weight are associated. Not only may there be a unifying cause but also failure to alter insulin dosage in these circumstances may contribute to hypoglycaemia.

Cognitive impairment

The potential for diabetes to cause cognitive impairment has been well documented over recent years, particularly in type 2 diabetes, although the exact nature of the relationship is not fully clarified.[39] This occurs against the background of increasing prevalence of dementia with age.

A significantly increased risk of cognitive impairment was reported in elderly diabetic subjects compared with a control population,[9] and Croxson et al[40] reported that in comparison to subjects with normal glucose tolerance, those with known diabetes were more likely to have a low mental test score. Other studies have tended to find similar results.[41,42] For instance, a prospective study reported an association between diabetes and cognitive decline as measured by repeated neuropsychological testing.[42]

The studies in brittleness in the elderly have pointed to cognitive impairment as both a single and contributory factor to glycaemic instability in this age group. Poor diabetic control itself may lead to worsening cognition,[43] thus beginning a cycle of decline.

Whether the cognitive impairment is secondary to hypertension, macrovascular disease, diabetes per se or another cause is less relevant in this situation. However, its recognition as a potential contributor to poor diabetes control is vital, although this may not be easy particularly in the earlier stages of the disease process.

Depression

Depression is a common finding in the background elderly population, but importantly an increased prevalence of depression in the elderly individual with diabetes has been reported.[9,44,45] In addition to the psychiatric consequences, depression can have a negative impact on cognitive abilities as well as on the desire or ability to engage in the self-management of diabetes, and it can lead to problems such as anorexia. Depression itself has been shown to have an adverse effect on glucose control.[46] Depression presenting as pseudodementia must also be considered.

Social factors

The residence and social circumstances may be relevant, although patients have been found to live in a variety of circumstances. Social isolation can be important[14] but, conversely, patients may be living in institutional care and still be 'brittle'.[17] A change in circumstance, for instance a recent bereavement, may have occurred. Although some individuals may benefit from institutional care, this is not a 'cure all' as recently the care, or otherwise, of people with diabetes in residential or nursing homes has come under scrutiny.[11,21,38,47,48] With an ageing population and greater numbers in care homes, the potential problems in this area may become more acute, as recent data has shown that approximately 25% of residents may have diabetes.[49]

Investigations

Diabetologists and geriatricians do not routinely work closely together, although there are exceptions. However, for elderly people with brittle diabetes, such cooperation may be beneficial, as each brings their own particular expertise to the situation. Similarly, the venue for investigation and management may need to be the geriatric day hospital rather than the diabetes centre. Whatever the site, extra clinic time is usually needed.

Evaluation should include a detailed history and examination (Table 9.2). In the former, the areas discussed earlier must be considered in detail. For instance, a thorough nutritional assessment may be needed, including a food diary. Particular attention should be paid to drug therapy and identifying or excluding any other coexistent illnesses. A

Table 9.2 Evaluation of elderly 'brittle' patients

General history:
- Nutrition
- Drug therapy
- Coexistent illnesses
- Social history

Physical examination

Functional assessment:
- Barthel Index

Cognitive assessment:
- Mini-Mental State Examination
- Geriatric Depression Scale

Laboratory tests

Multi-disciplinary review

full social history is vital and information may be obtained from family, friends, general practitioner, home help or social worker where appropriate. Although deliberate manipulation of therapy is thought unusual in the elderly brittle patient (particularly as the sole cause of instability) it is possible and therefore any potential gain for the patient should be explored. A thorough physical examination is mandatory, including lying and standing blood pressure. Visual acuity measurement should be considered. Screening for retinopathy, foot ulcers and neuropathy should also obviously be performed.

In contrast to the younger patient, particular attention must be paid to the functional abilities of the patient. Formal functional assessment can be performed using validated tools such as the Barthel Index,[50] which examines activities of daily living, including feeding and mobility. Cognitive function should be assessed for example by using the Mini-Mental State Examination (MMSE),[51] and mood by a tool such as the Geriatric Depression Scale.[52]

As with younger brittle patients, a detailed review of insulin technique and monitoring is necessary. However, a home visit by the diabetes specialist nurse may give extra information, which is useful in investigating brittleness.

Targeted investigations, as with the younger person, should be performed. These will include relevant biochemical, haematological and radiological tests to exclude or confirm organic disease. However, unlike the young, multidisciplinary assessment may be required from other medical and paramedical personnel. Formal psychogeriatric review may be necessary as well as physiotherapy, occupational therapy or social work assessment.

Management

Management should be aimed at addressing any specific issues identified, but as there may be multiple factors contributing to instability, multiple interventions may also be needed.

It should be appreciated that self-management strategies in the elderly brittle patient often require intensive input from the patient and therefore the patients' abilities are critically important. Specific management aims should include increasing the patients' understanding of diabetes through education, if possible. Diabetic patients over 65 have been shown to be more deficient than younger patients in knowledge of their condition[53] and there is reward to be gained in repetition and provision of written instructions. In cases where cognitive impairment exists, education of the carer must be embarked upon. Education and training of professionals caring for residents is also required.[11,21,54]

Management of the diabetes itself should include a review of insulin type, dosage, injection device, etc., as in any age group. Targets for metabolic control must always be individualized, but this is particularly important in the aged. It may be necessary to involve district nurses for injections, or to use short-acting analogue insulins after meals to optimize insulin dose adjustment. Insulin pumps have been advocated by some people for the elderly,[55,56] although they are not widely used.[57] Nutritional support may be necessary. Co-morbidities such as underlying arthritis, Parkinson's disease and stroke disease should be specifically addressed where possible, and functional aids may be needed. Other organic disease will need appropriate treatment, including depression when present. Cognitive impairment must be recognized and the appropriate strategies for management implemented where and when necessary, depending on individual circumstances. Psychogeriatric expertise may obviously be needed.

Further access to services may be beneficial. In the socially isolated patient having difficulty with meal preparation, the provision of a meals on wheels service or attendance at a day centre for lunch may provide a partial solution.

In all these cases a multi-agency, multidisciplinary approach is often necessary, including both diabetes and geriatric medicine teams.

Conclusions

Brittle diabetes has been shown to be present in the elderly. With the continuing ageing of the population, the rising prevalence of diabetes and the increasing use of insulin in this age group, the problems are likely to get worse. More work is needed to examine the prevalence of life-disrupting glycaemic instability in the elderly, and to determine the different mechanisms and aetiology from those found in the young. The often multifactorial aetiology requires a multidisciplinary approach between a variety of agencies, with access available to both diabetologists and geriatricians.

References

1. Census 2001. First results on population in England and Wales. The Stationary Office (TSO), 2002.

2. Croxson SCM, Burden AC, Bodington M, Botha JL. The prevalence of diabetes in elderly people. Diabet Med 1991; 8: 28–31.
3. Simmons D, William DR, Powel MJ. Prevalence of diabetes in a predominantly Asian community: preliminary findings of the Coventry diabetes study. Br Med J 1989; 298: 18–21.
4. Gatling W, Budd S, Walters D et al. Evidence of an increasing prevalence of diagnosed diabetes mellitus in the Poole area from 1983 to 1996. Diabet Med 1998; 15: 1015–21.
5. Drivsholm T, Ibsen H, Schroll M et al. Increasing prevalence of diabetes mellitus and impaired glucose tolerance among 60-year-old Danes. Diabet Med 2001; 18: 126–32.
6. Kilvert A, FitzGerald MG, Wright AD, Nattrass M. Newly diagnosed, insulin-dependent diabetes mellitus in elderly patients. Diabet Med 1984; 1: 115–18.
7. Sturrock NDC, Page SR, Clarke P, Tattersall RB. Insulin dependent diabetes in nonagenarians. Br Med J 1995; 310: 1117–18.
8. Mølbak AG, Christau B, Marner B et al. Incidence of insulin-dependent diabetes mellitus in age groups over 30 years in Denmark. Diabet Med 1994; 11: 650–5.
9. Dornan TL, Peck GM, Dow JDC, Tattersall RB. A community survey of diabetes in the elderly. Diabet Med 1992; 9: 860–5.
10. Tattersall RB. Diabetes in the elderly – a neglected area? Diabetologia 1984; 27: 167–73.
11. Croxson S. Diabetes in the elderly: problems of care and service provision. Diabet Med 2002; 19(suppl. 4): 66–72.
12. Gill GV. Does brittle diabetes exist? In: Gill GV, Pickup JC, Williams G, eds., Difficult diabetes. Blackwell Science, Oxford, 2001, pp 151–167.
13. Gale EAM, Dornan TL, Tattersall RB. Severely uncontrolled diabetes in the over-fifties. Diabetologia 1981; 21: 25–8.
14. Chapman J, Wright AD, Nattrass M, FitzGerald MG. Recurrent diabetic ketoacidosis. Diabet Med 1988; 5: 659–61.
15. Griffith DNW, Yudkin JS. Brittle diabetes in the elderly. Diabet Med 1989; 6: 440–3.
16. Gill GV, Lucas S, Kent LA. Prevalence and characteristics of brittle diabetes in Britain. Q J Med 1996; 89: 839–43.
17. Benbow SJ, Walsh A, Gill GV. Brittle diabetes in the elderly. J Roy Soc Med 2001; 94: 578–80.
18. Gill GV. The spectrum of brittle diabetes. J Roy Soc Med 1992; 85: 259–61.
19. Schade DS, Burge MR. Brittle diabetes: etiology and treatment. Adv Endocrinol Metab 1995; 6: 289–319.
20. Modawal A, Rudawsky DJ. 'Brittle' diabetes: the challenges of living with self-management strategies. J Am Geriatr Soc 2001; 49: S16–17.
21. Benbow SJ, Walsh A, Gill GV. Diabetes in institutionalised elderly people: a forgotten population? Br Med J 1997; 314: 1868–9.

22. Malone ML, Gennis V, Goodwin JS. Characteristics of diabetic ketoacidosis in older versus younger adults. J Am Geriatr Soc 1992; 40: 1100–4.
23. McAulay V, Frier BM. Hypoglycaemia. In: Sinclair AJ, Finucane P, eds., Diabetes in old age 2nd edn. John Wiley, Chichester, 2001, pp 133–52.
24. Meneilly GS, Cheung E, Tuokko H. Altered responses to hypoglycemia of healthy elderly people. J Clin Endocrinol Metab 1994; 78: 1341–8.
25. Brierly EJ, Broughton DL, James OFW, Alberti KGMM. Reduced awareness of hypoglycaemia in the elderly despite an intact counter-regulatory response. Q J Med 1995; 88: 439–45.
26. Jaap AJ, Jones GC, McCrimmon RJ et al. Perceived symptoms of hypoglycaemia in elderly Type 2 diabetic patients treated with insulin. Diabet Med 1998; 15: 398–401.
27. Thomson FJ, Masson EA, Leeming JT, Boulton AJM. Lack of knowledge of symptoms of hypoglycaemia by elderly diabetic patients. Age & Ageing 1991; 20: 404–6.
28. Matkya K, Evans M, Lomas J et al. Altered hierarchy of protective responses against severe hypoglycaemia in normal aging in healthy men. Diabetes Care 1997; 20: 135–41.
29. Frier BM, Fisher BM. Impaired hypoglycaemia awareness. In: Frier BM, Fisher BM, eds, Hypoglycaemia in clinical diabetes. John Wiley, Chichester, 1999, pp 111–46.
30. Damsgaard EM, Frøland A, Green A. Use of hospital services by elderly diabetics: the Frederica Study of diabetic and fasting hyperglycaemic patients aged 60–74 years. Diabet Med 1987; 4: 317–21.
31. Morgan CLl, Currie CJ, Stott NCH et al. The prevalence of multiple diabetes-related complications. Diabet Med 2000; 17: 146–51.
32. Tayal SC, Bansal SK, Chadha DK. Hypopituitarism; a difficult diagnosis in elderly people but worth a search. Age & Ageing 1994; 23: 320–2.
33. Fox RA. Diseases of the small bowel. In: Brocklehurst JC, Tallis RC, Fillit HM, eds., Textbook of geriatric medicine and gerontology, 4th edn. Churchill Livingstone, Edinburgh, 1992, pp 562–8.
34. Gregg EW, Beckles GLA, Williamson DF et al. Diabetes and physical disability among older U.S. adults. Diabetes Care 2000; 23: 1272–7.
35. Gregg EW, Mangione CM, Cauley JA et al. Diabetes and incidence of functional disability in older women. Diabetes Care 2002; 25: 61–7.
36. Lehmann AB. Undernutrition in elderly people. Age & Ageing 1989; 18: 339–53.
37. Caughey P, Seaman CEA, Parry DA et al. Dietary intake in the elderly estimated by a 24 hour recall and a food frequency questionnaire. J Hum Nutr Dietet 1994; 7: 209–13.
38. Benbow SJ, Hoyte R, Gill GV. Institutional dietary provision for diabetic patients. Q J Med 2001; 94: 27–30.
39. Gregg EW, Engelgau MM, Narayan V. Complications of diabetes in elderly people. Br Med J 2002; 325: 916–17.

40. Croxson SCM, Jagger C. Diabetes and cognitive impairment: a community-based study of elderly subjects. Age & Ageing 1995; 24: 421–4.

41. Ott A, Stolk RP, Hofman A et al. Association of diabetes mellitus and dementia: the Rotterdam Study. Diabetologia 1996; 39: 1392–7.

42. Fontbonne A, Berr C, Ducimetiere P, Alperovitch A. Changes in cognitive abilities over a 4-year period are unfavourably affected in elderly diabetic subjects. Diabetes Care 2001; 24: 366–70.

43. Gradman TJ, Laws A, Thompson LW, Reaven GM. Verbal learning and/or memory improves with glycemic control in older subjects with non-insulin-dependent diabetes mellitus. J Am Geriatr Soc 1993; 41: 1305–12.

44. Naliboff BD, Rosenthal M. Effects of age on complications in adult onset diabetes. J Am Geriatr Soc 1989; 37: 838–42.

45. Palinkas LA, Barrett-Connor E, Wingard DL. Type 2 diabetes and depressive symptoms in older adults: a population-based study. Diabet Med 1991; 8: 532–9.

46. Mazze RG, Lucido D, Shamoon H. Psychological and social correlates of glycemic control. Diabetes Care 1984; 7: 360–6.

47. Sinclair AJ, Allard I, Bayer A. Observations of diabetes care in long-term institutional settings with measures of cognitive function and dependency. Diabetes Care 1997; 20: 778–84.

48. Douek IF, Bowman C, Croxson S. A survey of diabetes management in nursing homes: the need for whole systems of care. Pract Diab Int 2001; 18: 152–4.

49. Sinclair AJ, Gadsby R, Penfold S et al. Prevalence of diabetes in care home residents. Diabetes Care 2001; 24: 1066–8.

50. Mahoney FI, Barthel DW. Functional evaluation: the Barthel Index. Maryland State Med J 1965; 14: 61–5.

51. Folstein MF, Folstein SE, McHugh PR. 'Mini-Mental State': a practical method for grading the cognitive state of patients for the clinician. J Psychiatr Res 1975; 12: 189–98.

52. Yesavage JA. Geriatric Depression Scale. Psychopharmacol Bull 1988; 24: 709–11.

53. Knight PV, Cummins AG, Kesson CM. Elderly diabetics: a case for education. J Clin Exp Gerontology 1983; 5: 285–94.

54. Guidelines of Practice for Residents with Diabetes in Care Homes. British Diabetic Association, London, 1999.

55. Rizvi AA, Petry R, Arnold MB, Chakraborty M. Beneficial effects of continuous subcutaneous infusion in older patients with long-standing Type 1 diabetes. Endocr Pract 2001; 7: 364–9.

56. Kamoi K. Good long-term quality of life without diabetic complications with 20 years of continuous subcutaneous insulin infusion therapy in a brittle diabetic elderly patient. Diabetes Care 2002; 25: 402–3.

57. Egger M, Davey Smith G, Stettler C, Diem P. Risk of adverse effects of intensified treatment in insulin-dependent diabetes mellitus: a meta-analysis. Diabet Med 1997; 14: 919–28.

chapter 10

The poorly controlled type 2 diabetic patient

Jon Pinkney and John Wilding

Poorly controlled type 2 diabetes is the single biggest challenge facing clinicians treating diabetes. Many patients with type 2 diabetes remain at high risk of complications, and so 'poor control' is simply defined as a failure to reach the recommended glycaemic and cardiovascular treatment targets. The scale of the problem is surprising after two decades of major advances in our knowledge of this disease and its treatment. Here we examine the extent of the problem, its causes and consider what can be done. Since poor control is often associated with obesity, we also consider the question, how should the obese patient with poorly controlled type 2 diabetes be treated?

Definitions and prevalence of poor glycaemic control

There are no glycaemic thresholds for diabetic complications. There is a straight line relationship between mean concentrations of glycated haemoglobin (HbA$_{1c}$) and diabetes-related end points (Fig. 10.1).[1] Therefore, any definitions of poor glycaemic control are arbitrary. Since poorly controlled diabetes is usually asymptomatic, a biochemical definition is necessary, such as a failure to reach agreed treatment

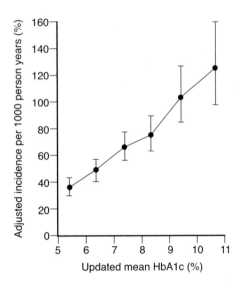

Figure 10.1 *Relationship between mean concentrations of glycated haemoglobin (HbA$_{1c}$) and incidence of diabetes-related complications in the UKPDS. Data are incidence rate and 95% confidence intervals by category of mean updated HbA$_{1c}$ adjusted for age, sex and ethnic group for white males aged 50–54 at diagnosis, and with mean duration of diabetes of 10 years. (Reproduced with permission of BMJ Publishing Group from Stratton et al, Br Med J 2000; 321: 405–12).*[1]

targets. European guidelines suggest HbA$_{1c}$ <6.5% as a definition for good control, whereas values >7.5% indicate poor control.[2] More recently, the American Diabetes Association (ADA) suggested HbA$_{1c}$ <7.0% as the target for satisfactory control, whereas HbA$_{1c}$ >8.0% requires action.[3] In support of these definitions, the risk of micro-vascular events with conventional treatment in the United Kingdom Prospective Diabetes Study (UKPDS) (mean HbA1c = 7.9%) was 11.4 events per 1000 patient-years versus 8.6 in the intensive treatment group (mean HbA$_{1c}$ = 7.0%) – 32% excess risk in the conventionally treated group.[4] Currently, however, non-alignment of HbA$_{1c}$ assays is a practical obstacle to widespread use of these definitions.

What proportion of patients with type 2 diabetes have HbA$_{1c}$ >7.0%? In recent reports from community and hospital studies in different countries, typical median HbA_{1c} values (using a variety of different assays) varied between 7.9 and 8.6%, with upper quartiles often around 10%.[5–9] In a recent audit of 800 patients with type 2 diabetes attending our hospital clinic in Liverpool, mean HbA_{1c} was 6.9% in diet-treated patients, 8.5% in those receiving oral hypoglycaemic drugs and 9.5% in those treated with insulin. Fifty-six per cent had an HbA_{1c} >8.1% and only 19% had an HbA1c <7.0% (unpublished data). An HbA_{1c} >10% indicates very poor control, often with symptoms, and usually erodes quality of life (QOL). Whatever the definition, poor glycaemic control is very common; using a definition of an HbA_{1c} >8.0%, in most populations it remains the rule.

The implications of poor glycaemic control are serious for patients and diabetes services alike. An important finding of the UKPDS was that each 1% decrement in mean HbA_{1c} reduced the risk of microvascular disease by 35% and diabetes-related deaths by 25%.[4] For those with retinopathy, a 1% reduction in mean HbA_{1c} over 10 years produced a 29% reduction in the risk of requiring laser photocoagulation and a 16% reduction in the risk of blindness in one eye.[4] The elderly and young need special mention. At the age of 70 years, average life expectancy in the UK is at least another 12 years for men and 15 for women (Department of Health: *www.doh.gov.uk/HPSSS/*) – plenty of time to develop serious microvascular disease. Therefore, it is inexcusable to deny elderly patients the benefits of good control. Lastly, childhood type 2 diabetes, common in many countries,[10] is now occurring in the UK.[11] These young people require the same lifelong intensive support as their peers with type 1 diabetes.

Causes and management of poor glycaemic control

A variety of factors explain the inability of most patients to achieve HbA_{1c} <7.0%. One underlying problem is that glycaemic control deteriorates with time, and this may explain why, after 9 years of follow-up, only 9%, 24% and 28% of patients treated by diet, sulphonylurea and insulin monotherapy, respectively, maintained HbA$_{1c}$ levels below 7.0% in the UKPDS.[12] Similar findings were found in the NHANES (National Health and Nutrition Examination Survey) III study.[13] This probably results from gradual deterioration of β-cell function.[14] Against this backdrop, we consider the impacts on glycaemic control of different aspects of management, environment and behaviour. Obesity cuts across all of these issues.

Dietary factors

Diet is first-line treatment and, in general, diet-treated patients, who are earlier in the natural history of diabetes, enjoy better glycaemic control. Nevertheless, the percentage of diet-treated patients with an HbA$_{1c}$ <7.0% was only 71% in NHANES III.[13] Inadequate control in diet-treated patients questions the efficacy of dietary and behavioural counselling and patient compliance, and suggests drug therapy is delayed too long. The most common dietary recommendations are for low saturated fat, low salt and high fibre, and, when weight loss is required, an energy deficit of up to 500 calories per day. However, weight loss is usually required, and sustained caloric restriction is essential if metabolic improvements are to be maintained. The difficulty is that this requires long-term behavioural change, and behavioural and lifestyle issues are usually not addressed adequately by conventional dietary consultations. Physical activity can also make a valuable contribution. Physical inactivity, reported by 50% of men with type 2 diabetes, was associated with a doubling of mortality over 12 years (Fig. 10.2).[15] Furthermore, a meta-analysis of 14 trials of exercise found that physical activity reduced average HbA$_{1c}$ levels by 0.6%.[16] It is harder to promote behavioural change than to prescribe drugs, but many patients with poor control would benefit from more frequent dietetic support and help in increasing physical activity rather than additional drug treatment.

Social and behavioural factors in poor glycaemic control

Social, behavioural and environmental factors exert major influences on glycaemic control. Mortality in people with type 2 diabetes is

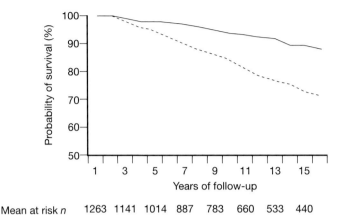

Figure 10.2 *Effect of physical fitness on all-cause mortality in patients with type 2 diabetes. Data are from 1263 men with 180 deaths during 14 777 man-years of observation. Physically fit men (solid line) had improved survival compared with unfit men (dashed line). (Reproduced with permission of American College of Physicians from Wei et al, Ann Intern Med 2000; 132: 605–11.[15])*

greater in those of lower social class, lower educational achievement and in those unemployed or living in council housing.[17] Presumably, educational and economic disadvantage are associated with reduced access to specialist care.[18] Disadvantaged patients need greater support in order to rectify poor glycaemic control. There is some evidence also that disordered eating is relatively common. Disinhibited eating is associated with higher body mass index (BMI),[19] and in one study the prevalence of binge eating was reportedly as high as 25%.[20] Smoking is more prevalent in lower socioeconomic groups and it is known that smoking is associated with insulin resistance and is an important risk factor for complications; interestingly, smoking cessation improves glycaemic control.[21] Although the risks of type 2 diabetes are increased in regular drinkers,[22] the impact of mild-to-moderate drinking on glycaemic control is rather less clear. Nevertheless, there is evidence that high alcohol consumption is associated with poorer dietary and therapeutic compliance.[23] However, light-to-moderate alcohol intake has the same cardioprotective effect in patients with diabetes as in those without.[24] In contrast, heavy alcohol intake has disruptive effects on diet and compliance and can be a big factor in poor glycaemic control.

In summary, for patients with inadequate glycaemic control it is essential to evaluate the social and behavioural background and adherence to previous advice regarding diet and physical activity.

Oral hypoglycaemic drugs

There are few long-term data comparing sulphonylureas, metformin, acarbose, glitinides and thiazolidinediones (TZDs), although trials of single agents versus placebo suggest similar short-term efficacies. Poor control remains common despite oral monotherapy and so combination therapies and insulin are frequently required. However, the optimum combinations of drugs are not well defined.

Despite treatment with sulphonylureas, many patients fail to reach HbA$_{1c}$ targets.[12,13] For example, in the intensive sulphonylurea-treated group of the UKPDS, 53% of patients also required insulin to maintain the glycaemic target.[25] Secondly, in overweight patients poorly controlled by diet, metformin is clearly superior to sulphonylureas or insulin in terms of diabetes-related end points and all-cause mortality.[26] Given the conservative (WHO) definition of obesity used in this study (BMI >30 kg/m^2), it is possible, but unproven, that metformin is also an appropriate first drug for many patients with lower levels of BMI, perhaps down to 25 kg/m^2.

Gradual weight gain is often seen in patients who are inadequately controlled. Many patients are obese at diagnosis and further weight gain is clearly undesirable. In UKPDS,[4] patients gained between 2.5 kg (diet-treated) and about 7.5 kg (insulin-treated) over 10 years. It is often inferred from this that weight gain is an expected part of the natural history of diabetes and ageing. One reason for favouring metformin as the first drug for obese patients is its weight-sparing effect.[27] For patients treated with insulin, the addition of metformin reduces weight gain by around 50%. In contrast to the UKPDS, however, a primary care study from Denmark has shown that modest weight loss is possible for type 2 patients; this result underlines the importance of dietetic and behavioural support and early use of metformin in obese patients.[28] Clearly, poor dietary support and prescribing – for example, first-line use of sulphonylureas in the obese, or insulin without metformin – can contribute to weight gain. The use of metformin even earlier in the natural history of the disease, as examined in the Diabetes Prevention Program,[29] could slow the decline in β-cell function and maintain euglycaemia for longer. Other drugs to consider, which might have less effect on weight than standard sulphonylureas are glitinides and glimepiride. It is also worthwhile remembering that body weight is increased by β blockers, tricyclic antidepressants, and some antipsychotics – especially clozapine and olanzapine.

Much interest has been generated by thiazolidinediones in the treatment of diabetes because of their effect on insulin sensitivity. In addition to the evidence that TZDs are effective as monotherapy[30] or add-on therapy,[31] they have been used successfully in 'triple therapy' with metformin and sulphonylureas,[32] and have been shown to improve glycaemic control and exert insulin-sparing effects when used with insulin.[33,34] However, TZDs are not licenced currently in Europe for 'triple therapy' or with insulin, and their long-term effects are uncertain.[35] Neither is the place of TZDs in treating obese patients well defined. TZDs improve insulin sensitivity but increase weight as a result of fluid retention and increased fat mass. TZDs promote subcutaneous fat deposition at the expense of visceral fat.[36] In a recent small uncontrolled study of severely obese insulin-treated-type patients, rosiglitazone significantly improved glycaemic control and allowed a 23% insulin dose reduction, despite a 3 kg weight increase.[37] At present, however, the principal use of TZDs in Europe is as add-on therapy for patients with poor control on other single agents.

It is clear also that non-compliance with advice and drug therapy are widespread. Non-compliance is partly related to polypharmacy, which is becoming the rule in type 2 diabetes.[38] In Denmark, around 70% of diabetic patients were prescribed at least 2 drugs, and the odds ratio for major polypharmacy (defined as 5 or more drugs) was 1.7 in diabetic patients.[39] It is essential to ascertain compliance before burdening patients with extra drugs.

Treatment with insulin

When oral therapy fails, there is usually no alternative to insulin. Whenever possible, it is also wise to continue metformin, as discussed above. However, poor glycaemic control can persist despite insulin. This was observed in both the UKPDS and NHANES III studies.[12,13] The reasons are complex and, in addition to the natural history of the disease, include difficulties with insulin administration, poor dietary adherence, patients' and carers' fears of hypoglycaemia (particularly the elderly) and unpredictable pharmacokinetics of some insulins. Procrastination in the use of insulin remains common; delays can arise because of reluctance by physicians or patients and families.

A common concern is that intensive treatment with insulin in people with type 2 diabetes will impair QOL. Is there any evidence for this? Encouragingly, QOL in the UKPDS was determined by the presence of complications and not by intensive treatment.[40] Likewise, in two other studies insulin had no negative effect on QOL.[41,42] However, other investigators have observed some impairment of QOL.[43] Interestingly, in the Fremantle study, QOL was well maintained immediately after insulin conversion, but declined after 1–2 years suggesting that insulin becomes onerous for some.[44] Once insulin is commenced, however, there seems little difference in QOL between patients treated with multiple injections or treated less intensively.[45] Given the hazards of poor glycaemic control, these data clearly support intensive treatment whenever possible, although sensitivity to QOL implications remains necessary. Insulin can be problematic in the frail elderly, in whom hypoglycaemia is a concern. In this group it often makes sense to accept less-stringent glycaemic control to maintain QOL rather than delay complications. It is possible that long-acting analogues such as insulin glargine may enable more patients to reach glycaemic targets with once-daily injections without increased risks of hypoglycaemia.[46] Inhaled insulin is another strategy that may allow more patients to achieve better control without injections.

Weight gain as a result of insulin treatment[4] is another frequent concern of patients and carers. The mechanism of insulin-induced weight gain remains controversial, although reduced metabolic rate and glycosuria are involved.[27] The peripheral anabolic action of insulin in adipose tissue may also override the satiety-promoting effects, leading to weight gain.[47] Although not well defined, weight gain may be most likely to occur in patients with poor dietary compliance, emphasizing the importance of education if insulin is to be successful.

Patients at high risk of cardiovascular disease

Cardiovascular disease (CVD) is common in people with type 2 diabetes[48] and its prevention is a major treatment objective. Individuals with high CVD risk can be identified by their clinical and biochemical characteristics.

Primary prevention of cardiovascular disease
The risk of CVD can be approached from the perspective of individual risk factors or calculations of aggregate risk. The two approaches are complementary. While severe dyslipidaemia and hypertension pose clear risks, risk scores identify many with less marked abnormalities who are also at high risk. Several methods have been devised to calculate CVD risk. Currently, the most widely used method in the United Kingdom is risk calculation based upon Framingham data, which is widely available as a convenient set of tables. However, it should be noted that these data are thought to underestimate risk in diabetic patients, for whom, it has been argued, CVD risk approaches that observed in non-diabetic patients who have had previous CVD events.

Treatment of dyslipidaemia
Most patients with type 2 diabetes have relatively modest lipid abnormalities – mildly reduced HDL (high-density lipoprotein) cholesterol, hypertriglyceridaemia, and normal or mildly elevated LDL (low-density lipoprotein) cholesterol (Fig. 10.3).[49] However, the implications become clear when aggregate CVD risk is calculated. Risk calculation has been advocated to guide treatment of dyslipidaemia and is widely

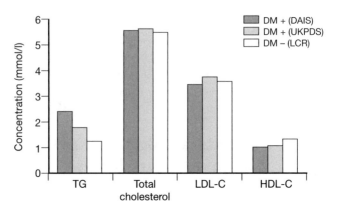

Figure 10.3 *Lipid profiles of patients with type 2 diabetes at entry to United Kingdom Prospective Diabetes Study (UKPDS), illustrating the modest nature of the defects. Comparison of baseline levels of triglycerides (TG), total cholesterol, low-density lipoprotein cholesterol (LDL-C), and high-density lipoprotein cholesterol (HDL-C) in patients with (+) and without (–) diabetes mellitus (DM) in the Diabetes Atherosclerosis Intervention Study (DAIS), UKPDS and the Lipid Research Council (LRC) Population Prevalence Study. (Reproduced with permission from UKPDS 27, Diabetes Care 1997; 20: 1683–7.[49])*

used in the UK.[50] In contrast, the ADA[51] and Joint European Task Force on Coronary Prevention[52] guidelines have emphasized lipid thresholds requiring action and treatment targets. The Joint European Task Force on Coronary Prevention in 1998 recommended treatment goals for total cholesterol <5.0 mmol/l (190 mg/dl) or LDL cholesterol <3.0 mmol/l (115 mg/dl).[52] The 2002 ADA recommendations advocated drug therapy for primary prevention at LDL cholesterol >3.35 mmol/l (130 mg/dl) and a treatment target <2.6 mmol/l (100 mg/dl).[51] Results from the Heart Protection Study support this approach. This study included a primary prevention cohort of 3982 diabetic patients with random LDL cholesterol >3.5 mmol/l (135 mg/dl) who were randomized to receive either simvastatin 40 mg or placebo. Over 5 years there was 26% reduction in CVD events in the simvastatin group.[53] One potential weakness of this approach is that no account is taken of HDL cholesterol. Levels of HDL cholesterol in the lowest tertile carry twice the coronary risk of levels in

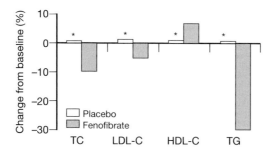

Figure 10.4 *Impact of treatment with micronized fenofibrate on dyslipidaemia in patients with type 2 diabetes in the Diabetes Atherosclerosis Intervention Study (DAIS) trial. HDL-C = high-density lipoprotein cholesterol; LDL-C = low-density lipoprotein cholesterol; TC = total cholesterol; TG = triglycerides; * = p<0.001. (Reproduced with permission from the Lancet 2001; 357: 905–10.[55])*

the upper tertile,[54] and the ADA recommend fibrate therapy for HDL <1.0 mmol/l (40 mg/dl) with LDL cholesterol in the range 2.6–3.3 mmol/l (100–129 mg/dl). Recent evidence suggests that fibrate therapy largely corrects the dyslipidaemia of diabetes and produces regression of coronary atheroma in type 2 diabetic patients (Fig. 10.4).[55] In this study, average levels of LDL and HDL cholesterol at baseline were just 3.4 and 1.0 mmol/l, respectively.

Theoretically, the risk score or lipid level for intervention ought to depend on the cost–benefit ratio, and this varies with age. Although cost–benefit is arbitrary, it has been suggested that lipid-lowering drugs are beneficial with 10-year risk >11% under the age of 30 years and >41% over the age of 80 years.[56] For type 2 diabetes it may be sensible to concentrate on those at highest risk (>20% 10-year risk). The cost-effectiveness of lipid-lowering therapy in patients with lower 10-year risks is more controversial.

Whether risk scores or lipid thresholds are used to manage dyslipidaemia, it is essential to identify high-risk patients by annual screening. Random lipid measurements are usually adequate, whereas insistence on fasting measurements usually means that some patients are not tested. Finally, failure to titrate drug doses to achieve lipid targets remains a widespread cause of persisting dyslipidaemia.

Poorly controlled blood pressure

Poorly controlled hypertension is common. The majority of people with type 2 diabetes are hypertensive – approximately 40–45% of patients in the UKPDS had blood pressures >160/90 at entry.[57] In another survey 78% of secondary and 55% of primary care patients had blood pressures >140/90.[58] In a recent survey in Liverpool we found that 62% of hospital patients and 75% of community patients with type 2 diabetes had blood pressures >140/85, and 45% of hospital patients and 49% of community patients with blood pressure above this level were not treated.[59] The risks from uncontrolled hypertension are serious, but are substantially reduced by effective treatment. Every 10 mmHg fall in blood pressure results in reductions of 12% in diabetes-related complications and 15% in diabetes-related deaths.[60] In the intensive blood pressure treatment group of UKPDS, in which blood pressure averaged 142/88, compared with 154/87 in the less-intensively treated arm, there was a 32% risk reduction for diabetes-related deaths after 9 years (Fig.

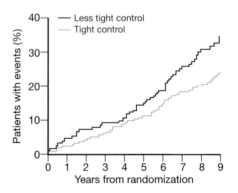

Reduction in risk with tight control 32% (95% CI 6% to 51%) (*P*=0.019)

Figure 10.5 *Impact of tight blood pressure control (averaging 142/82) versus less tight control (averaging 154/87) on diabetes-related deaths. Data are Kaplan–Meier plots of proportions of patients who die of diseases related to diabetes (myocardial infarction, sudden death, stroke, peripheral vascular disease and renal failure). (Reproduced with permission of BMJ Publishing Group from UKPDS 38, Br Med J 1998; 317: 703–13.[60])*

10.5).[60] The British Hypertension Society (BHS) guidelines recommended an optimal blood pressure of <140/80 in people with diabetes.[61] Recently, the ADA recommended initiation of drug therapy for blood pressure >140/90, with a goal of <130/80.[62]

Although such targets are clearly unrealistic for many – some experience the side effects of polypharmacy or unacceptable postural symptoms well before blood pressure reaches these ambitious levels – the strong relationship between blood pressure and risk argues that blood pressure should be reduced as much as possible. Frequent measurement of blood pressure is essential – infrequent appointments or poor attendance seriously impede this process. Our own experience suggests that blood pressure targets can be reached in up to 80% of patients in a dedicated nurse-led clinic, using algorithms to adjust therapy and add extra drugs as necessary.[59] Home and ambulatory monitoring are important back-up tools for diagnosis in borderline cases and to exclude white coat hypertension, and are useful in the assessment of difficult hypertension. If ambulatory blood pressure fails to respond to three or more drugs despite compliance, other causes of hypertension should be considered, including renal artery stenosis (RAS) – which is common in diabetes. An autopsy study found that about half of patients with RAS had type 2 diabetes, while the prevalence of RAS in hypertensive diabetic subjects was around 10%.[63] An investigation of type 2 diabetic patients with difficult hypertension also found that 16% had RAS.[64] Having excluded RAS, however, a high proportion of patients still require multiple antihypertensive drugs. In order to achieve blood pressures of <150/85, at least two antihypertensives were required by 60% of patients.[60] Clearly, the majority of patients are likely to need antihypertensive drugs to control CVD risk. There is also a strong case that one of the drugs should be an ACE (angiotensin-converting enzyme) inhibitor or angiotensin receptor antagonist.[65,66]

The patient who continues to smoke

The single most important objective for anyone with diabetes who smokes is to stop. Mortality from CVD is increased 10-fold in women who smoke; smoking cessation reduces this risk by 24% after 2 years,

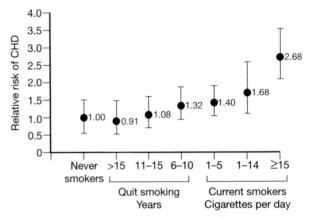

Figure 10.6 *Impact of current and previous smoking habits on coronary heart disease (CHD) in women with diabetes. Data are multivariate-adjusted relative risks of CHD. Vertical bars are 95% confidence intervals. (Reproduced with permission from Al-Delaimy et al, Arch Intern Med 2002; 162: 273–9.[68])*

but risk only approaches that of non-smokers after at least 10 years of abstinence.[67] In women with type 2 diabetes there is a surprising dose–response effect, and the risk of CVD is increased even in light smokers of just 1–5 cigarettes per day (Fig. 10.6). In diabetic smokers of >15 per day the risk of CVD was 7.7-fold increased compared with diabetics who had never smoked.[68] Diabetes and smoking are major, interacting risk factors for critical limb ischaemia and gangrene.[69] In people with diabetes the risk of major below-knee amputation is about 10-fold increased, and digital amputation a remarkable 400-fold increased.[70] Unfortunately, smoking cessation probably has limited impact on established critical limb ischaemia.

Smoking cessation is probably the most effective single step that can be taken to reduce CVD risk. It was estimated that smoking cessation increases life expectancy by about 3 years for a 45-year-old man with diabetes.[71] Although many patients worry about the weight gain of 2–4 kg that often follows smoking cessation[72] – and about 10% of people can gain in excess of 13 kg – the potential reduction in CVD risk far outweighs the metabolic harm from weight gain. Anti-smoking therapy and exercise can offset this weight gain. Although drugs such as bupropion and nicotine can facilitate smoking cessation,[73] they have not been evaluated in detail in people with diabetes. In the absence of serious coronary disease, however, the benefits may outweigh any theoretical risks.

The patient with microalbuminuria

In type 2 diabetes, microalbuminuria predicts the development of nephropathy and CVD[74] and is a useful indicator of CVD risk. Prospective studies showed that microalbuminuria increases CVD risk about 1.8-fold.[75] The association of microalbuminuria with CVD may be explained by its associations with hypertension and insulin resistance[76] and vascular endothelial dysfunction.[77] The presence of microalbuminuria identifies individuals who need aggressive control of risk factors for CVD. This approach has been shown to reduce macrovascular and microvascular events by around 50% compared with conventional treatment based on current guidelines.[77a]

The use of aspirin in patients with diabetes

The Hypertension Optimal Treatment (HOT) study[78] and the Early Treatment Diabetic Retinopathy Study[79] showed that regular treatment with aspirin reduced myocardial infarction by 17% and 15%, respectively. The doses used were 75 mg/day and 650 mg/day, respectively – thus, 75 mg is an appropriate dose for diabetic patients. Aspirin is still underused in patients with diabetes, and patients at high CVD risk should take aspirin unless there is a contraindication. For patients unable to tolerate aspirin, clopidogrel is an alternative.[80]

Secondary prevention of cardiovascular disease

The diabetic patients at highest risk of CVD are those with a history of myocardial infarction (Fig. 10.7), who have 40–50% mortality by 4–5 years[81,82] – about twice the rate of non-diabetic subjects. This is due to a high incidence of cardiac failure[83] and reinfarction.[84] Poor glycaemic control around the time of infarction increases mortality,[85] and it has been demonstrated that tight glycaemic control using

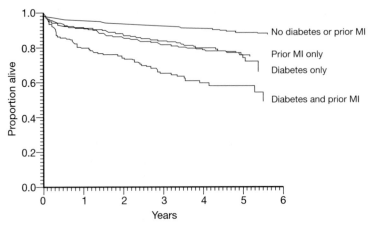

Figure 10.7 *Kaplan–Meier survival estimates after acute myocardial infarction (MI) according to presence of diabetes and prior MI. The curves for patients with only a prior MI or diabetes were both significantly different from the curves for patients with neither or both conditions (log-rank test for all comparisons, p <0.001). (Copyright © 2001 American Diabetes Association. Reproduced with permission from the American Diabetes Association, from Mukumal et al. Diabetes Care 2001; 24: 1422–7.[81])*

insulin, commenced at the time of infarction, reduces long-term mortality by 25%.[86] Other important aspects of secondary prevention for patients with type 2 diabetes include lipid lowering,[87] the early use of ACE inhibitors, aspirin and smoking cessation.

The obese patient with poorly controlled type 2 diabetes

Unfortunately, there is no simple answer to the question: 'What level of obesity is harmful for a patient with type 2 diabetes?' because the risk is continuous, and depends on fat distribution and other risk factors. Obesity is an independent risk factor for coronary heart disease in patients with type 2 diabetes.[88] Risk rises with increasing weight, whereas weight loss improves life expectancy.[89,90] However, BMI gives a poor estimate of body fat and is unrelated to fat distribution; therefore, the conventional definition of BMI >30 kg/m^2 for obesity is arbitrary and poorly related to the risks of diabetes and its complications. Those who would benefit most from weight loss may be better identified by waist circumference and lipid profiles,[91] although this has not yet been explored in detail in people with diabetes. Waist circumferences of 88–90 cm in women and 100–102 cm in men have been suggested as action levels that identify individuals who should lose weight.[91,92] Nevertheless, the association between obesity and diabetes is already apparent at BMI 25 kg/m^2 in most populations, and so many people with poorly controlled type 2 diabetes and BMI <30 kg/m^2 would benefit from weight loss. Once BMI is >30 kg/m^2, in the face of poor control, it is important to consider weight control as part of the overall treatment plan.

In theory, weight loss is an ideal treatment for type 2 diabetes. In 1986 Robert Henry and colleagues reported that weight loss averaging 16.8 kg in obese sulphonylurea-treated type 2 patients, weighing 103 kg at baseline, largely restored plasma glucose and hepatic insulin sensitivity to normal.[93] Nearly two decades later, what are the prospects for realizing weight loss of this magnitude more frequently in clinical practice?

Dietary and behavioural strategies

If an obese patient with poorly controlled type 2 diabetes wishes to lose weight much motivation is required. Without this, there is little point in proceeding further. A meta-analysis of clinical studies of different approaches to weight loss in patients with type 2 diabetes shows that dietary-based treatments are efficacious for weight loss and improving glycaemic control.[94] As usual, however, such good outcomes are more elusive in clinical practice, where there are many more patients and far fewer resources. Here, experience suggests that preaching occasional dietary advice to obese patients with diabetes has little impact. Besides self-motivation, people who want to achieve and maintain weight loss require encouragement, frequent and long-term contact and a detailed treatment plan that addresses behavioural issues, dietary content and physical activity. The potential efficacy of dietary-

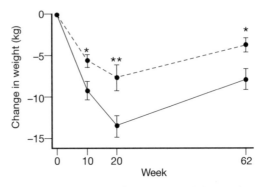

Figure 10.8 *Impact of the addition of exercise to a behavioural weight loss programme for obese type 2 diabetics. Changes in mean (SEM) weight at week 10, 20 and 62 for patients treated with diet alone (dashed line) and diet plus exercise (solid line). *p<0.01, **p <0.001. (Reproduced with permission of Springer-Verlag GmbH & Co. KG from Wing et al, Diabetologia 1988; 31: 902–9.[95])*

based behavioural strategies, particularly when combined with exercise programmes, in bringing about weight loss and improving glycaemic control has been confirmed (Fig. 10.8).[95] However, the main barrier to more widespread use of these strategies is that only a minority of people respond particularly well. For example, in a 12-month study Wing and colleagues[96] found that only about 24% of people were able to lose >6.9 kg or >5% weight – an amount that led to significant improvement in HbA1. Although weight loss >13.6 kg radically improved HbA1, few people in this study were able to achieve this degree of weight loss. It has also been suggested that diabetic patients treated with diet or oral drug therapy can lose weight as well as non-diabetic subjects but they have greater difficulty in maintaining the weight loss.[97] These findings draw attention to the need for improved strategies for both weight loss and relapse prevention. Lastly, however, a note of caution is struck by one interesting study of the impact of dietary-induced weight loss of at least 9.1 kg on glycaemic control in 135 obese diabetic patients. It was found that 41% of patients could be classed as 'responders', with significantly improved glycaemic control, whereas the remaining 59% still exhibited poor glycaemic control.[98] One interpretation of this is that patients with predominant insulin secretory failure may fail to benefit from weight loss to the same extent as those with predominant insulin resistance.

Another possible approach to weight loss in obese diabetic patients is partial dietary substitution with solid or liquid meal replacements (e.g. Slim-Fast™ foods). One or two meals are typically substituted with meal replacements, leaving a single healthy conventional meal in place, providing a total of about 1200–1400 calories daily. This approach achieves a greater energy deficit than standard low calorie diets, without the potential hazards of very low calorie diets (VLCD; see below), and may be useful for patients who have difficulty controlling portion size. Using this approach, it is necessary for patients with diabetes to monitor glycaemic control regularly in order to make any necessary reductions in oral hypoglycaemic drug or insulin doses. Meal replacement products have recently been used in combination with sibutramine and found to improve both weight loss and glycaemic control compared with standard therapy.[98a]

Very low calorie diets

Intensified dietary treatment using VLCD (400–800 cal/day), with or without meal replacements, is another approach that can produce substantial short-term metabolic improvements in patients with diabetes. However, in view of the previously suggested risk of sudden death associated with rapid and severe weight loss, caused perhaps by cardiac protein malnutrition and arrhythmias,[99] this approach should only be used for short periods under expert supervision. The main use of these approaches is to achieve rapid weight loss, although in less intense and intermittent forms they have been used for more extended periods. Table 10.1 summarizes some of the VLCD and meal replacement studies in obese diabetic patients. Many patients showed near-normalization of blood glucose, blood pressure and lipids, and large reductions in insulin doses, and occasionally insulin withdrawal was reported. These data are concordant with the results of bariatric surgery.[100] Although the data show that aggressive caloric restriction is highly beneficial in the short term, the prevention of long-term relapse remains a problem. In a recent VLCD study with meal replacements

Table 10.1 Weight loss studies in patients with type 2 diabetes that have involved the use of a very low calorie diet (VLCD) with or without meal replacements

Authors	N	Duration (weeks)	Mean weight at entry (kg)	Weight loss (kg)	Daily energy intake (Cal)	Comments	Ref
Hanefeld and Weck	29	4	84.7	10	290–335	Major reductions in glucose, lipids and blood pressure	117
Di Biase et al	12	5–8	119	14.6	330	'Cambridge diet'. Blood glucose became normal by day 4. Another 14 patients were unable to tolerate the diet	118
Wing et al	18	20	102.1	18.6	400	VLCD+ BT. Major metabolic improvement. No difference in weight loss from standard BT at 1 year	119
Rotella et al	29	2	82.9	10.6	450	30% fall in FBG. Study included 16 insulin-treated subjects. Major falls in insulin doses, and insulin withdrawn in one subject	120

Smith and Wing	45	12	103.9	16.3	400–500	Metabolic data not reported. Weight loss was much less (1.42 kg) during a second period of VLCD	103
Wing et al	93	50		14.2	400–500	RCT of VLCD versus LCD	121
Capstick et al	14	12	108.9	94.5	425	Significant falls in HbA_{1c}, lipids and blood pressure, insulin	122
Williams et al	54	20	104	10	400–600	RCT of 2 periodic VLCD regimens versus BT. Intermittent 5-day VLCD most effective method. Improved glycaemic control in both VLCD groups compared with BT	123

BT = behavioural therapy, FBG = fasting blood glucose, RCT = randomized controlled trial.

in obese type 2 patients, long-term weight loss was less well maintained than by those who followed a conventional LCD.[101] Attention has been drawn to the difficulties in complying with hypocaloric diets[102] and the tendency for diminished compliance with repeated attempts to lose weight.[103] Therefore, an intensively supervised, short-duration VLCD can be effective for rapid weight loss, but if this approach is to find wider acceptance better strategies are needed to prevent relapse. Despite these problems, it is hard not to point out the similarity between obesity and other chronic diseases such as hypertension, asthma, arthritis and some cancers. Many of these diseases relapse if treatment is withdrawn. Relapse is not a legitimate argument against helping obese people with diabetes to lose weight.

Role of antiobesity drugs

Antiobesity drugs can help to prevent or reduce relapse in the maintenance phase of weight loss programmes.[104] The role of these drugs, however, in patients with diabetes is not well defined. Table 10.2 summarizes published studies of orlistat and sibutramine – the two principal antiobesity drugs available – in type 2 diabetes. Few other drugs, past or present, have been studied in large numbers of patients with diabetes, although there is some evidence that fluoxetine,[105,106] and prior to its withdrawal fenfluramine[107,108] and the combination of fenfluramine and phentermine[109] had similar effects. Short-term data suggest that orlistat and sibutramine are moderately effective in maintaining weight loss in patients with diabetes.[110,111] However, in a multicentre randomized controlled trial (RCT) in which 550 obese insulin-treated patients were randomized to receive orlistat or placebo for 52 weeks, the orlistat group only lost about 2.6 kg more than the placebo group, with small but significant improvements in glycaemic control.[112] In this study, patient support – a critical component – was not particularly intensive, and other aspects of treatment influence weight change in diabetic patients. The magnitude of these effects makes it unlikely that antiobesity drugs will have a major impact in the diabetes clinic without additional measures. The foremost question is whether the combination of more structured,

Table 10.2 Trials of antiobesity drugs orlistat and sibutramine in patients with type 2 diabetes

Authors	N	Drug	Duration	Initial weight (kg)	Weight loss (kg) vs placebo	Comments	Ref
Hollander et al	391	Orlistat	1 year	99	−2.4	RCT. 49% on orlistat lost >5% body weight vs 23% on placebo. 0.46% group difference in HbA$_{1c}$. Small improvements in lipids	110
Kelley et al	550	Orlistat	1 year	102	−2.6	RCT. Study of insulin-treated patients. −0.35% fall in HbA$_{1c}$ in orlistat group. Small reductions in diabetes therapy and lipid improvements	112
Fujioka et al	175	Sibutramine	24 weeks	99	−3.9	RCT. 0.4 kg loss in placebo group. 33% patients lost >5% weight; 8% patients lost >10% weight. >5% weight loss ~ 0.5% HbA$_{1c}$ fall. Small lipid improvements	124
Finer et al	91	Sibutramine	12 weeks	84	−2.3	RCT. 19% sibutramine patients lost >5% weight, vs 0% with placebo. 0.3% fall in HbA$_{1c}$ in sibutramine group vs 0% with placebo	111
Gokcel et al	60	Sibutramine	6 months	95	−8.7	RCT. Unusually poor response in placebo group. −2.2% fall in HbA$_{1c}$ with sibutramine. Improved lipids and insulin sensitivity	125

RCT = randomized controlled trial.

supervised dietary and behavioural modifications together with antiobesity drugs in the maintenance phase would be more effective? Thus, antiobesity drugs can, in principle, be used in conjunction with meal replacements, or following short periods of VLCD. Given resources, intensive support and motivation, some obese diabetic patients do well with weight loss and derive considerable metabolic benefit. Currently, however, it looks unrealistic that this form of treatment could be offered on a wide scale. A recent survey of dietetic services for people with diabetes in the UK[113] suggests that there are too few dietitians for obesity to receive sufficient attention.

Bariatric surgery in type 2 diabetes

If weight loss and metabolic improvements are not forthcoming with other methods, another potential approach is bariatric surgery. The operations currently performed include gastric restrictive procedures (gastric banding and gastroplasty) and combined gastric restrictive and malabsorption procedures (gastric bypass, biliopancreatic diversion). Gastric restrictive procedures are usually performed laparoscopically, and malabsorption procedures can also be performed in this way. This field has been reviewed in detail.[114] Although specific trials in patients with diabetes are lacking, the available data suggest that reductions in therapy, withdrawal of tablets or insulin, and sometimes full remission of diabetes occur frequently. There are also some rather tantalizing data from a non-randomized and retrospective study which suggested that bariatric surgery might reduce mortality in morbidly obese diabetic patients.[115] It has been suggested that bariatric surgery is worth considering for diabetic patients with BMI >35 kg/m^2,[116] although in our own hospital clinic about 25% of type 2 diabetic patients fall into this category (unpublished observation). Table 10.3 summarizes the reported effects of bariatric surgery in patients with type 2 diabetes; there are also considerable improvements in QOL. However, none of these data are randomized, and long-term RCTs in obese patients with type 2 diabetes are still needed to define which operations are best, and which patients might benefit from these procedures as the primary approach to controlling the diabetes.

Table 10.3 Impact of bariatric surgery on medical treatment requirements for type 2 diabetes

Authors	N	Surgery	Follow-up interval	Weight loss	Preoperative treatment for diabetes	Postoperative treatment for diabetes	Ref
Herbst et al	23	Various	20 months	27.2 kg	Insulin $n = 23$	Insulin $n = 7$, plus major dose. Reductions in $n = 6$	126
Brolin	21	GBP	12 months	N/S	Insulin $n = 21$	Insulin $n = 7$	127
MacGregor and Rand	12	Various	3–13 years	N/S	Insulin $n = 10$	Insulin $n = 2$	128
Reinholt	N/S	GBP	5 years	N/S	Insulin/OHA 11.6%	Insulin/OHA 5.8%	129
Pories et al.	165	GBP	7.6 years	33%	N/S	83% 'remission'	130
Stieger et al	20	LGB	1 year	N/S	N/S	14/20 'remission'	131
Scheen	24	VBG	28 months	30 kg	Insulin/OHA $n = 7/22$	Insulin/OHA $n = 4/6$	132
Dixon and O'Brien	50	LGB	12 months	27 kg	Insulin/OHA $n = 4/29$	Insulin/OHA $n = 4/8$ 64% 'remission'	133
SOS	196	Various	2 years	28 kg	Insulin/OHA $n = 8/40$ Diet/no therapy $n = 70$	Insulin/OHA $n = 6/16$ Diet/no therapy $n = 86$	*
	77	Non-surgical	2 years	–	Insulin/OHA $n = 3/32$ Diet/no therapy $n = 42$	Insulin/OHA $n = 5/44$ Diet/no therapy $n = 26$	

GBP = gastric bypass, LGB = laparoscopic gastric banding, N/S = not stated, OHA = oral hypoglycaemic agent, VBG = vertical band gastroplasty, SOS = Swedish Obese Subjects study, *CD Sjöström, personal communication.

Conclusions

The patient with poorly controlled type 2 diabetes is at high risk and should be identified by screening and treated unambiguously to the agreed targets. Inadequate professional support and a variety of persisting patient behaviours usually contribute to poor control. Regular follow-up by an expert multidisciplinary diabetes team – not simply an annual review – is mandatory. A history of previous CVD events, a high CVD risk score, smoking and the presence of micro-albuminuria identify diabetic patients at particularly high risk. When relevant, smoking cessation is likely to result in the single biggest risk reduction. Aspirin also continues to be an underused primary preven-tion treatment. In general, intensive treatment does not have a negative effect on QOL, and good control is no less important in the elderly. Obesity is also a common and neglected factor: some patients enjoy large metabolic benefits from weight loss. Improved glycaemic control and CVD risk reduction are often evident with 5% weight loss and can be considerable with >10% weight loss. Motivated individu-als can do well; those lacking motivation rarely succeed. Intensive and long-term dietetic support with an emphasis on behavioural change is essential. For some patients short-term VLCD, with or without meal replacements, results in rapid weight loss, although relapse is common. Antiobesity drugs in the weight maintenance phase may help some patients. Above a BMI of 35 kg/m^2, however, it is worth considering bariatric surgery. Ideally, diabetes clinics ought to offer weight management programmes, at least for those patients motivated to pursue this approach.

References

1. Stratton IM, Adler AI, Neil AW et al. Association of glycaemia with macrovascular and microvascular complications of type 2 diabetes (UKPDS 35): prospective observational study. Br Med J 2000; 321: 405–12.
2. Alberti KG, Gries FA, Jervell J, Krans HM. A desktop guide for the

management of non-insulin dependent diabetes mellitus (NIDDM): an update. European NIDDM Policy Group. Diabet Med 1994; 11: 899–909.

3. American Diabetes Association. Position Statement. Standards of medical care for patients with diabetes mellitus. Diabetes Care 2002; 25(suppl 1): S33–49.

4. UKPDS Study Group. Intensive blood glucose control with sulphonylureas or insulin compared with conventional treatment and risk of complications in patients with type 2 diabetes (UKPDS 33). Lancet 1998; 352: 837–53.

5. Valle T, Koivisto VA, Reunanen A, Kangas T, Rissanen A. Glycemic control in patients with diabetes in Finland. Diabetes Care 1999; 22: 575–9.

6. Nicholls GA, Hillier TA, Javor K, Brown JB. Predictors of glycemic control in insulin-using adults with type 2 diabetes. Diabetes Care 2000; 23: 273–7.

7. Chan WB, Chan JCN, Chow CC et al. Glycaemic control in type 2 diabetes: the impact of body weight, β-cell function and patient education. Q J Med 2000; 93: 183–90.

8. Bruno G, Cavallo-Perin P, Bargero G et al. Glycaemic control and cardiovascular risk factors in type 2 diabetes: a population-based study. Diabet Med 1998; 4: 304–7.

9. Khunti K, Ganguli S, Baker R, Lowy A. Features of primary care associated with variations in process and outcome of care of people with diabetes. Br J Gen Pract 2001; 51: 356–60.

10. Rosenbloom AL, Joe JR, Young RS, Winter WE. Emerging epidemic of type 2 diabetes in youth. Diabetes Care 1999; 22: 345–54.

11. Drake AJ, Smith A, Betts PR, Crowne EC, Shiled JP. Type 2 diabetes in obese white children. Arch Dis Child 2002; 86: 207–8.

12. Turner RC, Cull CA, Frighi V, Holman RR. Glycemic control with diet, sulphonylurea, metformin, or insulin in patients with type 2 diabetes mellitus: progressive requirement for multiple therapies (UKPDS 49). J Am Med Assoc 1999; 281: 2005–12.

13. Shorr RI, Franse LV, Resnick HE et al. Glycemic control of older adults with type 2 diabetes: findings from the Third National Health and Nutrition Examination Survey, 1988–1994. J Am Geriatr Soc 2000; 48: 264–7.

14. DeFronzo RA, Bonadonna RC, Ferrannini E. Pathogenesis of NIDDM. A balanced overview. Diabetes Care 1992; 15: 318–68.

15. Wei M, Gibons LW, Kampert JB, Nichaman MZ, Blair SN. Low cardiorespiratory fitness and physical inactivity as predictors of mortality in men with type 2 diabetes. Ann Intern Med 2000; 132: 605–11.

16. Boulé NG, Haddad E, Kenny GP, Wells GA, Sigal RJ. Effects of exercise on glycemic control and body mass in type 2 diabetes mellitus. J Am Med Assoc 2001; 286: 1218–27.

17. Robinson N, Lloyd CE, Steven LK. Social deprivation and mortality in adults with diabetes mellitus. Diabet Med 1998; 15: 205–12.

18. Beckles GLA, Engelgau MM, Venkat Narayan KM et al. Polulation-based assessment of the level of care among adults with diabetes in the U.S. Diabetes Care 1998; 21: 1432–8.
19. Straub RH, Lamparter-Lang R, Palitzch KD, Scholmerich J. Association between eating behaviour and current glycaemic control, body mass or autonomic nervous function in long-term type I and type II diabetic patients. Eur J Clin Invest 1996; 26: 564–8.
20. Crow S, Kendall D, Praus B, Thuras P. Binge eating and other psychopathology in patients with type II diabetes. Int J Eat Disord 2001; 30: 222–6.
21. Gunton JE, Davies L, Wilmshurst E, Fulcher G, McElduff A. Cigarette smoking affects glycemic control in diabetes. Diabetes Care 2002; 24: 796–7.
22. Holbrook TL, Barrett-Connor E, Wingard DL. A prospective population-based study of alcohol use and non-insulin dependent diabetes mellitus. Am J Epidemiol 1990; 132: 902–9.
23. Johnson KH, Bazargan M, Bing EG. Alcohol consumption and compliance among inner-city minority patients with type 2 diabetes mellitus. Arch Fam Med 2000; 9: 964–70.
24. Ajani UA, Gaziano JM, Lotufo PA et al. Alcohol consumption and risk of coronary heart disease by diabetes status. Circulation 2000; 102: 500–5.
25. Wright A, Burden ACF, Paisey RB, Cull CA, Holman RR. Sulphonylurea inadequacy. Efficacy of addition of insulin over 6 years in patients with type 2 diabetes in the UK Prospective Diabetes Study (UKPDS 57). Diabetes Care 2002; 25: 330–6.
26. UKPDS Study Group. Effect of intensive blood glucose control with metformin on complications in overweight patients with type 2 diabetes (UKPDS 34). Lancet 1998; 352: 854–65.
27. Makimattila S, Nikkila K, Yki-Jarvinen H. Causes of weight gain during insulin therapy with and without metformin in patients with type II diabetes mellitus. Diabetologia 1999; 42: 406–12.
28. de Fine Olivarius N, Beck-Nielsen H, Helms Andreasen A, Horder M, Pedersen PA. Randomised controlled trial of structured personal care of type 2 diabetes mellitus. Br Med J 2001; 323: 970–5.
29. Knowler WC, Barrett-Connor E, Fowler SE et al. Reduction in the incidence of type 2 diabetes with lifestyle intervention or metformin. N Engl J Med 2002; 346: 393–403.
30. Phillips LS, Grunberger G, Miller E et al. Once- and twice-daily dosing with rosiglitazone improves glycemic control in patients with type 2 diabetes. Diabetes Care 2001; 24: 308–15.
31. Yale JF, Valiquett TR, Ghazzi MN et al. The effect of a thiazolidinedione drug, troglitazone, on glycemia in patients with type 2 diabetes mellitus poorly controlled with sulfonylurea and metformin. A multicenter,

randomized, double-blind, placebo-controlled trial. Ann Intern Med 2001; 134: 737–45.

32. Bell DS, Ovalle F. Long term efficacy of triple oral therapy for type 2 diabetes mellitus. Endocr Pract 2002; 8: 271–5.

33. Schwartz S, Raskin P, Fonseca V, Graveline JF. Effect of troglitazone in insulin-treated patients with type II diabetes mellitus. Troglitazone and Exogenous Insulin Study Group. N Engl J Med 1998; 338: 861–6.

34. Rosenstock J, Einhorn D, Hershon K, Glazer NB, Yu S. Pioglitazone 014 Study Group. Efficacy and safety of pioglitazone in type 2 diabetes: a randomised, placebo-controlled study in patients receiving stable insulin therpy. Int J Clin Pract 2002; 56: 251–7.

35. Krentz AJ, Bailey CJ, Melander A. Thiazolidinediones for type 2 diabetes. Br Med J 2000; 321: 252–3.

36. Mori Y, Murakawa Y, Okada K et al. Effects of troglitazone on body fat distribution in type 2 diabetic patients. Diabetes Care 1999; 22: 908–12.

37. Buch HN, Baskar V, Barton DM et al. Combination of insulin and thiazolidinedione therapy in massively obese patients with type 2 diabetes. Diabet Med 2002; 19: 572–4.

38. Veehof L, Stewart R, Haaijer-Ruskamp F, Meyboom-de Jong BM. The development of polypharmacy: a longitudinal study. Fam Pract 2000; 17: 261–7.

39. Bjerrum L, Sogaard J, Hallas J, Kragstrup J. Polypharmacy: correlations with sex, age and drug regimen. Eur J Clin Pharmacol 1998; 54: 197–202.

40. UK Prospective Diabetes Study Group. Quality of life in type 2 diabetic patients is affected by complications but not by intensive policies to improve blood glucose or blood pressure control (UKPDS 37). Diabetes Care 1999; 22: 1125–36.

41. de Grauw WJ, van de Lisdonk EH, van Gerwen WH, van den Hoogen HJ, van Weel C. Insulin therapy in poorly controlled type 2 diabetic patients: does it affect quality of life? Br J Gen Pract 2001; 51: 527–32.

42. de Sonnaville JJ, Snoek FJ, Colly LP et al. Well-being and symptoms in relation to insulin therapy in type 2 diabetes. Diabetes Care 1998; 21: 919–24.

43. Redekop WK, Koopmanschap MA, Stolk RP et al. Health-related quality of life and treatment satisfaction in Dutch patients with type 2 diabetes. Diabetes Care 2002; 25: 458–63.

44. Davis TM, Clifford RM, Davis WA. Effect of insulin therapy on quality of life in type 2 diabetes mellitus: the Fremantle Diabetes Study. Diabetes Res Clin Pract 2001; 52: 63–71.

45. Schiel R, Muller UA. Intensive or conventional insulin therapy in type 2 diabetic patient? A population-based study on metabolic control and quality of life (The JEVIN-trial). Exp Clin Endocrinol Diabetes 1999; 107: 506–11.

46. Yki-Jarvinen H, Dressler A, Ziemen M. Less nocturnal hypoglycaemia

and better post-dinner glucose control with bedtime insulin glargine compared with bedtime NPH insulin during insulin combination therapy in type 2 diabetes. Diabetes Care 2000; 23: 1130–6.

47. Schwartz MW, Woods SC, Porte D, Seeley RJ, Baskin DG. Central nervous system control of food intake. Nature 2000; 404: 661–71.

48. Kannel WB, McGee DL. Diabetes and cardiovascular disease: the Framingham Study. J Am Med Soc 1979; 241: 254–60.

49. UK Prospective Diabetes Study Group. UK Prospective Diabetes Study 27. Plasma lipids and lipoproteins at diagnosis of NIDDM by age and sex. Diabetes Care 1997; 20: 1683–7.

50. British Cardiac Society. Joint British recommendations on prevention of coronary heart disease in clinical practice. Heart 1998; 80: S1–29

51. American Diabetes Association. Management of dyslipidemia in adults with diabetes. Diabetes Care 2002; 25: S74–7.

52. Prevention of coronary heart disease in clinical practice. Recommendations of the Second Joint Task Force of European and other societies on coronary prevention. Eur Heart J 1998; 19: 1434–503.

53. Heart Protection Study Collaborative Group. MRC/BHF Heart Protection Study of cholesterol lowering with simvastatin in 20,536 high-risk individuals: a randomised placebo-controlled trial. Lancet 2002; 360: 7–22.

54. Turner RC, Millns H, Neil HAW et al. Risk factors for coronary artery disease in non-insulin dependent diabetes mellitus: United Kingdom prospective diabetes study (UKPDS: 23). Br Med J 1998; 316: 823–8.

55. Diabetes Atherosclerosis Intervention Study Investigators. Effect of fenofibrate on progression of coronary-artery disease in type 2 diabetes: the Diabetes Atherosclerosis Intervention Study, a randomised study. Lancet 2001; 357: 905–10.

56. van Hout BA, Simoons ML. Cost-effectiveness of HMG coenzyme reductase inhibitors; whom to treat? Eur Heart J 2001; 22: 751–61.

57. UKPDS Study Group. UKPDS III. Prevalence of hypertension and hypotensive therapy in patients with newly diagnosed diabetes. A multicentre study. Hypertension 1985; 7: II8–II13.

58. Moore WV, Fredrickson D, Brenner A et al. Prevalence of hypertension in patients with type II diabetes in referral versus primary care clinics. J Diab Comp 1998; 12: 302–6.

59. Woodward A, Groves T, Wallymahmed M, Wilding JP, Gill GV. Attaining UKPDS management targets in type 2 diabetes: failures and difficulties. Pract Diabet 2001; 18: 307–10.

60. UKPDS Study Group. Tight blood pressure control and risk of macrovascular and microvascular complications in type-2 diabetes: UKPDS 38. Br Med J 1998; 317: 703–13.

61. Ramsey LE, Williams B, Johnston GD et al. British Hypertension Society guidelines for hypertension management 1999: summary. Br Med J 1999; 319: 630–5.

62. American Diabetes Association. Treatment of hypertension in adults with diabetes. Diabetes Care 2002; 25: S71–3.
63. Sawicki P, Kaiser S, Heinemann L, Frenzel H, Berger M. Prevalence of renal artery stenosis in diabetes mellitus – an autopsy study. J Intern Med 1991; 229: 489–92.
64. Courreges JP, Bacha J, Aboud E, Pradier P. Prevalence of renal artery stenosis in type 2 diabetes. Diabetes Metab 2000; 26: 90–6.
65. Heart Outcomes Prevention Evaluation (HOPE) Study Investigators. Effects of ramipril on cardiovascular and microvascular outcomes in people with diabetes mellitus: results of the HOPE study and MICRO-HOPE substudy. Lancet 2000; 355: 253–9.
66. Lindholm LH, Ibsen H, Dahlof B et al. Cardiovascular morbidity and mortality in patients with diabetes in the Losartan Intervention for Endpoint reduction in hypertension study (LIFE); a randomised trial against atenolol. Lancet 2002; 359: 1004–10.
67. Kawachi I, Colditz GA, Stampfer MJ et al. Smoking cessation and time course of decreased risks of coronary heart disease in middle aged women. Arch Intern Med 1994; 154: 169–75.
68. Al-Delaimy WK, Manson JE, Solomon CG et al. Smoking and risk of coronary heart disease among women with type 2 diabetes mellitus. Arch Intern Med 2002; 162: 272–9.
69. Dormandy J, Heeck L, Vig S. Predicting which patients will develop chronic critical leg ischemia. Semin Vasc Surg 1999; 12: 138–41.
70. Humphrey LL, Palumbo PJ, Butters MA et al. The contribution of non-insulin dependent diabetes to lower extremity amputation in the community. Arch Intern Med 1994; 154: 885–92.
71. Yudkin JS. How can we best prolong life? Benefits of coronary risk factor reduction in non-diabetic and diabetic subjects. Br Med J 1993; 306: 1313–18.
72. Williamson DF, Madans J, Anda RF et al. Smoking cessation and severity of weight gain in a national cohort. N Engl J Med 1991; 324: 739–45.
73. Jorenby DE, Leischow SJ, Nides MA et al. A controlled trial of sustained release bupropion, a nicotine patch, or both for smoking cessation. N Engl J Med 1999; 340: 685–91.
74. Mogensen CE. Microalbuminuria predicts clinical proteinuria and early mortality in maturity-onset diabetes. N Engl J Med 1984; 310: 356–60.
75. Mattock MB, Barnes DJ, Viberti G-C et al. Microalbuminuria and coronary heart disease. Diabetes 1998; 47: 1786–92.
76. Groop L, Ekstrand A, Forsblom C et al. Insulin resistance, hypertension and microalbuminuria in patients with type 2 (non-insulin dependent) diabetes mellitus. Diabetologia 1993; 36: 642–7.
77. Stehouwer CD, Nauta JJ, Zeldenrust GC et al. Urinary albumin excretion, cardiovascular disease, and endothelial dysfunction in non-insulin-dependent diabetes mellitus. Lancet 1992; 340: 319–23.

77a. Gaede P, Vedel P, Larsen N, Jensen GVH, Parving H-H, Pedersen O. Multifactorial intervention and cardiovascular disease in patients with type 2 diabetes. N Engl J Med 2003; 348: 383–93.

78. HOT study group. Effects of intensive blood-pressure lowering and low dose aspirin in patients with hypertension: principal results of the Hypertension Optimal Treatment (HOT) randomised trial. Lancet 1998; 351: 1755–62.

79. ETDRS Investigators. Aspirin effects on mortality and morbidity in patients with diabetes mellitus. Early Treatment Diabetic Retinopathy Study report 14. J Am Med Assoc 1992; 268: 1292–300.

80. Creager MA. Results of the CAPRIE trial: efficacy and safety of clopidogrel. Clopidogrel versus aspirin in patients at risk of ischaemic events. Vasc Med 1998; 3: 257–60.

81. Mukumal KG, Nesto RW, Cohen MC et al. Impact of diabetes on long term survival after acute myocardial infarction. Comparability of risk with prior myocardial infarction. Diabetes Care 2001; 24: 1422–7.

82. Donnan PT, Bioyle DIR, Broomhall J et al. Prognosis following first acute myocardial infarction in type 2 diabetes: a comparative population study. Diabet Med 2002; 19: 448–55.

83. Abbott RD, Donahue RP, Kannel WB, Wilson PW. The impact of diabetes on survival following myocardial infarction in men versus women. The Framingham Study. J Am Med Assoc 1988; 260: 3456–60.

84. Haffner SM, Lehto S, Ronnemaa T, Pyorala K, Laaksu M. Mortality from coronary heart disease in subjects with type 2 diabetes and in non-diabetic subjects with and without prior myocardial infarction. N Engl J Med 1998; 339: 229–234.

85. Rytter L, Troelson S, Beck-Nielsen H. Prevalence and mortality of acute myocardial infarction in patients with diabetes. Diabetes Care 1985; 8: 230–4.

86. Malmberg K, Norhammar A, Wedel H, Ryden L. Glycometabolic state at admission: important risk marker of mortality in conventionally treated patients with diabetes mellitus and acute myocardial infarction: long-term results from the Diabetes and Insulin-Glucose Infusion in Acute Myocardial Infarction (DIGAMI) study. Circulation 1999; 99: 2626–32.

87. Scandinavian Simvastatin Survival Study group. Randomised trial of cholesterol lowering in 4444 patients with coronary heart disease: the Scandinavian Simvastatin Survival Study (4S). Lancet 1994; 344: 1383–9.

88. Cho E, Manson JE, Stampfer MJ et al. Obesity and the risks of heart disease in diabetes. Diabetes Care 2002; 25: 1142–8.

89. Lean MEJ, Powrie JK, Anderson AS. Obesity, weight loss and prognosis in type 2 diabetes. Diabet Med 1990; 7: 228–33.

90. Williamson DF, Thompson TJ, Thun M et al. Intentional weight loss and mortality among overweight individuals with diabetes. Diabetes Care 2000; 23: 1451–2.

91. Despres J-P, Lemieux I, Prud-homme D. Treatment of obesity: need to focus on high risk abdominally obese patients. Br Med J 2001; 322: 716–20.
92. Lean ME, Han TS, Morrison CE. Waist circumference as a measure for indicating need for weight management. Br Med J 1995; 311: 158–61.
93. Henry RR, Wallace P, Olefsky JM. Effects of weight loss on mechanisms of hyperglycaemia in obese non-insulin-dependent diabetes mellitus. Diabetes 1986; 35: 990–8.
94. Brown SA, Upchurch S, Anding R, Winter M, Ramirez G. Promoting weight loss in type II diabetes. Diabetes Care 1996; 19: 613–24.
95. Wing RR, Epstein LH, Paternostro-Bayles M et al. Exercise in a behavioral weight control programme for obese patients with type-2 (non-insulin dependent diabetes). Diabetologia 1988; 31: 902–9.
96. Wing RR, Koeske R, Epstein LH et al. Long term effects of modest weight loss in type II diabetic patients. Arch Intern Med 1987; 147: 1749–53.
97. Guare J, Wing R, Grant A. Comparison of obese NIDDM and non-diabetic women: short- and long-term weight loss. Obesity Res 1995; 3: 329–35.
98. Watts NB, Spanheimer RG, DiGirolamo M et al. Prediction of glucose response to weight loss in patients with non-insulin-dependent diabetes mellitus. Arch Intern Med 1990; 150: 803–6.
98a Redman JB, Raatz SK, Reck KP, Swanson JE, Kwong CA, Fan Q, Thomas W, Bantle JP. One year outcome of a combination of weight loss therapies in subjects with type 2 diabetes: a randomized trial. Diabetes Care 2003; 26: 2505–11.
99. Sours HE, Frattali VP, Brand D et al. Sudden death associated with very low calorie weight reduction regimes. Am J Clin Nutr 1981; 34: 453–61.
100. Pinkney JH, Sjöstrom CD, Gale EAM. Should surgeons treat diabetes in very obese people? Lancet 2001; 357: 1357–9.
101. Paisey RB, Frost J, Harvey P et al. Five year results of a prospective very low calorie diet or conventional weight loss programme in type 2 diabetes. J Hum Nutr Diet 2002; 15: 121–7.
102. Zilli F, Croci M, Tufano A, Caviezal F. The compliance of hypocaloric diet in type 2 diabetic obese patients: a brief-term study. Eat Weight Disord 2000; 5: 217–22.
103. Smith DE, Wing RR. Diminished weight loss and behavioural compliance during repeated diets in obese patients with type 2 diabetes. Health Psychol 1991; 10: 378–83.
104. Finer N, Finer S, Naoumova RP. Drug therapy after very-low-calorie diets. Am J Clin Nutr 1992; 56: 195S-8S.
105. Gray DS, Fujioka K, Devine D, Bray GA. Fluoxetine treatment of the obese diabetic. Int J Obes 1992; 16(suppl 4): 567–72.
106. Connolly VM, Gallagher A, Kesson CM. A study of fluoxetine in obese elderly patients with type 2 diabetes. Diabet Med 1995; 12: 416–18.
107. Stewart GO, Stein GR, Davis TM, Findlater P. Dexfenfluramine in type II diabetes: effect on weight and diabetic control. Med J Aust 1993; 158: 167–9.

108. Willey KA, Molyneaux LM, Overland JA, Yue DK. The effect of dexfen-fluramine on blood glucose control in patients with type 2 diabetes. Diabet Med 1992; 9: 341–3.

109. Redmon JB, Raatz SK, Kwong CA et al. Pharmacologic induction of weight loss to treat type 2 diabetes. Diabetes Care 1999; 22: 896–903.

110. Hollander PA, Elbein SC, Hirsch IB et al. Role of orlistat in the treatment of obese patients with type-2 diabetes. Diabetes Care 1998; 21: 1288–94.

111. Finer N, Bloom SR, Frost GS, Banks LM, Griffiths J. Sibutramine is effective for weight loss and diabetic control in obesity with type 2 diabetes: a randomised, double-blind, placebo-controlled study. Diabet Obes Metab 2000; 2: 105–12.

112. Kelley DE, Bray GA, Pi-Sunyer FX et al. Clinical efficacy of orlistat therapy in overweight and obese patients with insulin-treated type 2 diabetes. Diabetes Care 2002; 25: 1033–41.

113. Winocour PH, Mearing C, Ainsworth A, Williams DRR. Association of British Clinical Diabetologists (ABCD): survey of specialist diabetes care services in the UK, 2000. Dietetic services and nutritional issues. Diabet Med 2002; 19: 39–43.

114. Sjöström L. Surgical intervention as a strategy for the treatment of obesity. Endocrine 2001; 13: 213–30.

115. MacDonald KG, Long SD, Swanson MS et al. The gastric bypass operation reduces the progression and mortality of non-insulin dependent diabetes mellitus. J Gastrointestin Surg 1997; 1: 213–20.

116. National Institutes of Health Consensus Development Conference. Am J Clin Nutr 1992; 55: 487S-619S.

117. Hanefeld M, Weck M. Very low calorie diet therapy in obese non-insulin-dependent diabetes patients. Int J Obes 1989; 13(suppl 2): 33–7.

118. Di Biase G, Mattioli PL, Contaldo F, Mancini M. A very low calorie formula diet (Cambridge diet) for the treatment of diabetic-obese patients. Int J Obes 1981; 5: 319–24.

119. Wing RR, Marcus RD, Salata R et al. Effects of a very low calorie diet on long term glycemic control in obese type 2 diabetic subjects. Arch Intern Med 1991; 151: 1334–40.

120. Rotella CM, Cresci B, Mannucci E et al. Short cycles of very low calorie diet in the therapy of obese type II diabetes mellitus. J Endocrinol Invest 1994; 17: 171–9.

121. Wing RR, Blair E, Marcus M, Epstein LH, Harvey J. Year-long weight loss treatment for obese patients with type II diabetes: does including an intermittent very low calorie diet improve outcomes? Am J Med 1994; 97: 354–62.

122. Capstick F, Brooks BA, Burns CM et al. Very low calorie diet (VLCD): a useful alternative in the treatment of the obese NIDDM patient. Diabetes Res Clin Pract 1997; 36: 105–11.

123. Williams KV, Mullen ML, Kelley DE, Wing RR. The effect of short periods of caloric restriction on weight loss and glycemic control in type 2 diabetes. Diabetes Care 1998; 21: 2–8.

124. Fujioka K, Seaton TB, Rowe E et al. Weight loss with Sibutramine improves glycaemic control and other metabolic parameters in obese patients with type 2 diabetes mellitus. Diabetes Obes Metab 2000; 2: 175–87.

125. Gokcel A, Karakose H, Erteror EM et al. Effects of sibutramine in obese female subjects with type 2 diabetes and poor blood glucose control. Diabetes Care 2001; 24: 1957–60.

126. Herbst CA, Hughes TA, Gwynne TJ, Buckwalter JA. Gastric bariatric operation in insulin-treated adults. Surgery 1984; 95: 209–14.

127. Brolin RE. Results of obesity surgery. Gastroenterol Clin N Am 1987; 16: 317–38.

128. Macgregor AMC, Rand CSW. Gastric bypass in morbid obesity. Arch Surg 1993; 128: 1153–7.

129. Reinhold RB. Late results of gastric bypass surgery for morbid obesity. J Am Coll Nutr 1994; 13: 326–33.

130. Pories WJ, Swanson M, MacDonald KG et al. Who would have thought it? An operation proves to be the most effective therapy for adult onset diabetes mellitus. Ann Surg 1995; 222: 339–52.

131. Stieger R, Thurnbeer M, Lange J. Morbide obesitas: Ergebnisse des "laparoscopic gastric banding" bei 130 konsekutiven patienten. Schweiz Med Wochenschr 1998; 128: 1239–46.

132. Scheen AJ. Aggressive weight reduction treatment in the management of type 2 diabetes. Diabetes and Metabolism 1998; 23: 116–23.

133. Dixon JB, O'Brien PE. Health outcomes of severely obese type 2 diabetic subjects 1 year after laparoscopic adjustable gastric banding. Diabetes Care 2002; 25: 358–63.

chapter 11

Psychological intervention for brittle diabetes

Jackie Fosbury

Introduction

In the past few years clinicians have begun to recognize the importance of psychological factors in diabetes management and diabetes control. This recognition has finally transferred into more psychologically orientated recommendations for diabetes care, most recently for example within the British Government's National Service Framework (NSF) for diabetes.[1]

In part, recognition of the importance of psychological factors in diabetes care has lain within a final acceptance that, for many patients, long-term diabetes education and medical investigations have not improved people's ability or willingness to be self-caring.

In fact, much of the success of the US Diabetes Control and Complications Trial (DCCT) is attributed to the psychological care offered to patients during the study.[2]

Psychological research has focused around measuring the *difficulties* that could affect diabetes management and control and render education ineffective. Once the prevalence of these variables was established, we began to research the various psychological *treatments* that may improve these difficulties. In a recent paper, Snoek and Skinner reported on the five common psychological problems known to complicate diabetes management, and they reviewed research into the effects of psychological treatments.[3]

Very little psychological research has been conducted in 'brittle' diabetes however, although treatments have been reviewed in patients exhibiting 'self-destructive behaviours'.[4] This is defined by high glycated haemoglobin (HbAlc) levels, recurrent diabetic ketoacidosis (DKA) and/or severe recurrent hypoglycaemia. These symptoms are in fact components of what *some authors* refer to as 'brittleness'. In this chapter 'brittleness' is seen as the outcome of psychological processes. In addition, psychological treatment research, which has widely used cognitive behavioural therapy (CBT), has focused on 'mono-symptomatic' presentations in diabetes (e.g. depression). Brittle diabetes, however, is a multi-symptomatic medical *and psychological* presentation. Erratic glycaemic control, frequent hospitalization and the *seeming impossibility* of control on standard insulin systems can be 'fed' by a multiplicity of underlying causes, e.g. disordered eating, depression, anxiety and/or neurotic difficulties. Ryle's[5] definition of neurotic behaviour is when someone continues to act in ways that work badly for them, but they are unable to revise their ideas or behaviour in the light of adverse outcomes. This behaviour produces harmful or restricting results, which do not get revised. 'Neurotic' individuals are often characterized by deficient or costly patterns of self-care and by failures of mutuality in relation to others.

This chapter outlines the history and casework of cognitive analytic therapy (CAT), developed by Ryle[5] in what could be defined as a 'brittle' patient. CAT has been used as part of a psychotherapy diabetes service at St Thomas' and Guy's hospitals in London for 12 years. The CAT service is used for a wide range of psychological and emotional presentations in diabetes, and is continuously audited both in terms of glycaemic and psychological well-being. The arrangement of this service is being used as a blueprint for services in other UK diabetes centres. It will be argued that complex psychodynamic treatments (such as CAT) are the therapy of choice in diabetes as they 'emphasize the underlying motivations of behaviour and processes of change and development'.[6] CAT has developed techniques and treatment for understanding and intervening in complex presentations such as 'brittle' diabetes or self-destructive behaviours.

History of the service

As with many diabetes services, the centres at Guy's and St Thomas' hospitals offer a full psychologically orientated programme of diabetes education to their patients. The aim was to seek to maximize the patient's capacity for effective and autonomous control of their diabetes. However, despite this programme, a substantial proportion of attending patients persisted with poor glycaemic control (HbA$_{1c}$ >10.0%). Many of these patients were frequently hospitalized in an attempt at stabilization. It was of course recognized that an inner-city teaching hospital would draw a high number of complex patients and cases.

The nursing staff and dieticians, who had good psychological skills and relationships with patients, were also skilled enough to recognize that their abilities were different from those required for actual psychological treatment methods. In particular, they continued to point out that these patients with long-term poor control actually had very good diabetes knowledge but did not blood test, rarely took their insulin regularly and never considered their diet. This meant that their consultations were not only 'unproductive' but they were often 'overused'.[7] This meant that their diabetes education was also expensive.

This state of affairs led clinicians to approach the Psychotherapy Department to initiate a research enquiry in the Diabetes Unit at St Thomas' Hospital into any psychological problems their patients may have with their diabetes. Initially, Jane Milton, a psychoanalyst interviewed a number of type 1 and type 2 diabetes patients with persistent poor control.[8] Her interviews revealed that a number of psychological and emotional issues would affect a person's ability or willingness for self-care and glycaemic stability. Many of these patients 'preferred' to be admitted to hospital rather than stay at home.

As a result of Milton's work, a randomized controlled intervention study of CAT was conducted with long-term, poorly controlled type 1 patients.[9] Twenty-six patients were either randomized into intensive diabetes nurse specialist education, or to CAT. The important outcome in this work was that the patients in the education group improved their glycaemic control during treatment but relapsed by 9 months of follow-up. The CAT group, however, did not improve their control until *after* their psychotherapy had ended, and this improvement continued to the 9-month retest point. On the basis of these results, and a clear freeing up of nursing and dietetic time, a full-time CAT service was funded to cover both diabetes sites.

Cognitive analytic therapy

Cognitive analytic therapy is a focused time-limited (normally 16 sessions) psychotherapy that combines techniques and understandings from psychoanalytic and cognitive behavioural therapy. It was developed by Ryle, and has a strong research base. It has been used successfully to treat a wide range of psychological disorders, covering deliberate self-harm,[10] grief and depression,[11] asthma[12] and borderline personality disorders.[13]

There are many ways in which CAT differs from CBT. One is fundamental – unlike CBT, the underlying theory in CAT is derived from psychoanalysis. Thus, there is a great deal of emphasis in CAT on the therapeutic relationship itself and early experiences (causation) are seen as central to the work. Damaging difficulties emanating from these early experiences will not only be the topic of therapeutic conversations but also they will be re-enacted (and interpreted and analysed) in the relationship of the patient to the therapist and to the tasks of the therapy. In particular, diabetic patients with chronic poor self-care and control are frequently, by definition, resistant to self-care, advice and treatment. Resistance is central to the work of psychoanalysis and central to helping people with chronic poor self care. If work with resistance is avoided, the essence of the therapy is avoided. Thus, Ryle and colleagues describe what happens if one works in a more cognitive, rational and educational way with patients, and one where the therapist avoids resistance:

> An approach which demands the rational cooperation of the patient, such as CBT, will often fail, especially in more disturbed patients, because the patient is uncooperative (resistant) – that is to say, the patient behaves in a way typical of his or her problem.[14]

CBT requires a cooperative, rational encounter with patients where self-monitoring and diary-keeping of negative thoughts and actions are elicited often around a particular goal, e.g. blood glucose monitoring, feelings of low self-esteem, etc. The theoretical approach is derived from behavioural psychology and is based on learning paradigms that seek to alter overt behaviour and feelings.[15] CAT, on the other hand, offers a comprehensive understanding of the nature of early unconscious self-destructive drives and functioning. Thus, a patient with 'brittle diabetes' usually does not present what they do or do not do (overt) in relation to their diabetes self-care. Trying to elicit this information is often redundant and would encounter more resistance! What they do embrace in therapy, however, is the patterning of early experiences and relationships, which may lead them to think and act against themselves and others.

CAT is based on a theoretical model related to the object relations (OR) school of psychoanalysis. This means that CAT emphasizes the origin of personality and patterns of relating (to self, self-care and others) in early childhood relationships with key, significant others (objects). Thus, a CAT therapist elicits information about the patient's early formative experiences/relationships and the impact and construction of these experiences and relationships on their current emotional and psychological difficulties and self-care procedures.

Early positive relationship information may reveal for example that the patient may have been an excited child to a stimulating parent, or a satisfied child to a providing parent. Alternatively, negative experiences may reveal a protesting child to a controlling parent, a deprived child to an abandoning parent and so forth. Eventually the theoretical model reveals that the child internalizes an understanding of two roles: one played by the self, which is referred to as the internal child-derived role (IC); and one by the parents or carers, the (IP) role. Hence, a version of the parental roles also becomes internalized and, in due course, the individual can play out not only his own role but also this other role, being able to enact either child-derived or parent-derived roles in subsequent relationships. This is referred to in CAT as a reciprocal role relationship (RRR). In diabetes work it is usual to uncover a number of these destructive relationship patterns configuring around diabetes management and control. They are most frequently – abusive to abused; neglecting to neglected; conditionally cared for to undermined and guilty; indifferent care to a child who feels worthless and empty; critical and undermining to a criticized, undermined, striving child.

These learnt parent-derived and child-derived roles are eventually re-enacted by the patients towards others and towards themselves, as in self-neglect and self-abuse. It would be very difficult to have good diabetes self-care with these early experiences as the foundation for life.

Confirmation of re-enactment is subsequently found within the patient's history of childhood experiences, schooling, work difficulties and current relationship issues. The re-enactment is also confirmed around diabetes self-care and the elicitation of poor care from others, e.g. frequency of being rejected and neglected by others (who give up on them or want to ideally rescue then disappoint them). This pattern would also include medical carers and psychologists. The re-enactment is often unconscious and needs to be made conscious during the therapy. The re-enactment is referred to as transference, i.e. transferring early experiences (e.g. of being rejected or wanting to reject) onto all other relationship situations.

Transference is a central concept in psychoanalytic work. It refers to the venting of positive (falling in love with, idealizing 'you are the perfect doctor/nurse/psychologist') and negative (contempt and wanting to destroy) past experiences, projected onto the therapist. The importance of the transference is that it allows the therapist to see *hidden* feelings and *denied* actions. This is very important in work with patients who often deny some of their diabetes actions. The therapist's job is to recognize the transference once it arises, and accept it uncritically, and then to interpret it and feed its origins back to the patient. This psychoanalytic stance ensures that the therapist and patient become fully involved in the painful and dangerous aspects of the work. The expectation of this negative transference will be mooted to the patient in the first or second sessions of the therapy. Milton describes the difference between CBT and CAT in this regard. The patient may constantly invite the therapist towards what she describes as a 'weak form of CBT – to be a nice therapist, to explain and reassure, but ultimately to be a weak transference object'.[16] The therapist's own therapy (which is a requirement to practice CAT and other psychoanalytic therapies) reduces the therapist's need to gratify the patient in this way and therefore increases the scope of dealing with destructive issues brought up in the therapy.

A unique feature of CAT is the emphasis on *reformulating* the patient's problems in the early sessions of the therapy. Reformulation is derived from the basis of early work with the patient, where an agreed written description of those negative and damaging modes of relating are outlined in letter form to the patient. The reformulation also includes the clearest possible description of the patient's harmful or ineffective procedures. The term 'procedure' refers to an individual's way of organizing aspects of their lives around aims, relationships and self-management. A full account of a procedure is of a circular, usually self-maintaining process. It will describe a regular sequence of mental processes, an account of the action and outcome. A 'neurotic' procedure is one which produces harmful results, which do not get revised. Three main patterns account for this failure to revise: they are called traps, dilemmas and snags.[5]

Traps

Traps are actions that we feel we cannot escape from: examples are avoidance, depressed thinking, social isolation and placation traps. In these situations, negative assumptions generate acts that produce consequences, which reinforce the assumptions. In the case of depressed thinking, we are sure we will manage a task or social situation badly. We are therefore not as effective as we could be, which leads us to exaggerate how badly we handled things, which makes us feel more depressed about ourselves. Placatory behaviour has its roots in feeling uncertain about ourselves. We are therefore anxious not to upset others. We therefore try to please people by doing what they seem to want. As a result we can end up being taken advantage of by others, which makes us angry, depressed or guilty – from which, our uncertainty about ourselves is confirmed. Sometimes we may feel out of control because of the need to please, and we start hiding away, putting things off, letting people down; this makes others feel angry with us, which increases our uncertainty. Trying to deal with feeling ineffective and anxious, depressed, underconfident or uncertain about ourselves will lead us to act in ways that confirm our fears, thereby resulting in a vicious circle, in which however hard we try things seem to get worse instead of better.

Dilemmas

Dilemmas are false choices and narrow options. They arise when we act or feel as *if* available actions or possible roles are limited to polarized alternatives (false dichotomies), usually without being aware that this is the case. Dilemmas are often clearly drawn from core parental experiences such as critical parent to criticized and undermined child. Thus a patient may play out 'either I am critical and undermining or criticized and undermined'. A common dilemma in diabetes work is around 'complying or defying': for example,

I feel as if looking after myself is submitting to others, and this makes me feel dependent, resentful and out of control; so I don't, I rebel, feel independent and free, but unwell.

Not surprisingly, this young patient was a frequent inpatient at the time, with this dilemma continuously being re-enacted.

Snags

Snags are the obstacles we face when we want to change: 'I want to change *but* ...'. Appropriate goals or roles are abandoned by patients either on the true or false assumption that others would oppose them, or independently of the views of others *as if* they were forbidden or dangerous. The individual may be more or less aware that she is acting in this way and may or may not relate this to feelings such as guilt if things go well for her. For example, in the case of a patient whose mother resented her relationship with her father and was very envious and critical of her, one snag was, 'If I look nice at work my colleagues won't like me' (e.g. fearing destructive envy via projecting her early experiences on to the work place). This patient would subsequently and frequently omit daily insulin, feeling full of self-disgust and loathing about the way she looked and also feeling that she could control something (albeit negatively) by that omission. She was also a frequent inpatient. Another example was, 'I cannot control my diabetes because my parents would feel useless.'[17]

CAT includes a number of paperwork tools to focus on problem procedures and revision within the time limit. The central tools are the prose reformulation letter, which outlines traps, snags and dilemmas, and a diagram which confirms the self-maintaining sequential nature of these traps, snags and dilemmas. Diagrams include a model of the patient's core state(s) in which the repertoire of reciprocal roles are listed and from which the various damaging procedures in the diabetic patient are generated. Diabetic procedures are concerned with relationships with others, self-care and the points at which self-care are sabotaged.

CAT can often circumvent these patterns through the process of joint reformulation, and will address the potentially life-threatening behaviours within an understanding of the reciprocal role repertoire. Once a patient gets to a position of not wanting to feel, think or act in damaging ways, discussion takes place as to possible alternatives or revision, where ineffective procedures are replaced with more adaptive ones. This is achieved both by the patient learning to recognize the operation of these procedures in their day-to-day lives or relationships through self-observation and by the therapist drawing attention to the manifestation of these procedures in the therapeutic relationship. Once recognition has occurred, effective new ways of being can be explored. *It is unlikely that trying to find solutions before the problems are accurately identified is likely to be successful.*

In understanding how therapy can change people, CAT draws on many sources, but the underlying assumption is that all therapies involve, in varying proportions, the patient's exposure to new experience, new behaviour, and new understanding. The change sought in CAT is procedural change, which includes the full range of perception, memory, judgement, planning action and evaluation. To do this the main focus in CAT is on the therapeutic relationship and on insight. The therapist needs to offer respecting care and, with the help of the reformulation, avoid responses that serve to reinforce the patient's damaging procedures. The success of short-term therapy depends on patients learning to know themselves accurately and, in respect of their main destructive tendencies, so that conscious thought can intervene to block and, in due course, replace damaging procedures.

Undertaking CAT with a self-destructive patient

June was a 25-year-old patient who had agreed to have her CAT taped for analysis. The transcripts have been analysed individually and have been presented in detail.[18] June was very typical of patients referred to the psychotherapy service. She had been diagnosed at 10 years old and had had poor control since she was 15 years old (HbA_{1c} on referral was 12.2%). June was referred by another hospital consultant. He described her as an 'unfortunate young girl' with recurrent

DKA and severe retinopathy. She also had a history of psychiatric intervention for 'depression', and local community mental health teams, including an art therapist, had been involved in her care since diagnosis. She was also described as 'unmotivated', with a history of considerable interpersonal and family difficulties.

When I saw June for her assessment, she described herself as 'not being bothered' about her diabetes or herself in general. She sometimes took insulin, never monitored blood glucose and ate what she wanted. In the past, she was a regular inpatient and denied not taking her insulin, but as she had her own flat away from her parents, she seemed less interested in being hospitalized now. She had constant pains in her feet, and also headaches, and in part this was the reason she decided to attend for therapy. She presented as virtually catatonic! June's history describes her internalized parent and child derived roles and how they are replayed with her diabetes.

History

June was very close to her mother but felt ignored and rejected when her older sister was present. As a response to this, she felt 'blanked out', as if she did not matter. June said she was very similar to her mother however, in so far as they were both walked all over (procedure). There was considerable conflict between June's parents due to her father's irresponsibility and unreliability. As a consequence, June felt let down and resentful towards her father. This made her feel as if she could not be bothered with people and herself, and so she internalized the father's role as someone who modelled forms of unreliable and irresponsible care. He could also be stubborn. June described herself as feeling 'real hate' towards her father because of the way in which 'he makes mum feel'.

When June was diagnosed as having diabetes everything seemed to change. She received a lot of active attention from her parents. Her father became reliable and attentive and her mother stopped ignoring her, but eventually this drove June 'mad'. She felt as if she only mattered because of her diabetes. Being so angry with her parents but feeling as if she could not express it, she turned the anger

243

in against herself. 'If they bother, why should I?' This *dilemma* replicated itself with many of June's subsequent carers and was interpreted in her therapy. Eventually, however, people stopped bothering with June – they blanked her out (because she was unreliable, irresponsible, stubborn and ignoring).

The problem then was that June found she was unable to care for herself consistently and reliably. Feeling second best in relation to her sister (ignoring and rejecting to ignored and rejected), and receiving unreliable irresponsible care from her father, gave June no psychological equipment with which to relate to others positively, elicit care from others or to care for herself. Her *traps* were:

1. Feeling blanked out, as if I don't matter, I try and let others care for me, but if they bother, I don't, so they get resentful, ignore and reject me so I feel blanked out
2. I try and care for others but feel easily walked all over, so I think why should I? I become stroppy and unreliable and let them down, so they get angry, reject and ignore me
3. Feeling I don't matter, I feel hurt and angry but can't express it, so I just hurt myself

June's diagram is shown in Figure 11.1.

Transference issues

During the initial stages of the therapy June was virtually monosyllabic, blanking out most of the work, but was stubborn enough to attend. Her presence 'felt' stroppy and was interpreted as possible anger and resentment that she was in the room because of her diabetes. But there was also a sense of hurt, which had to be expressed – that she could be ignored to the effect that she felt as if she did not matter. She presented herself as if she did not matter, and people treated her as such. Blanking out the sessions could in fact lead me to feel that she was not bothered about them, and I might feel as if I wanted to not bother with her, and that was presented to June in the room.

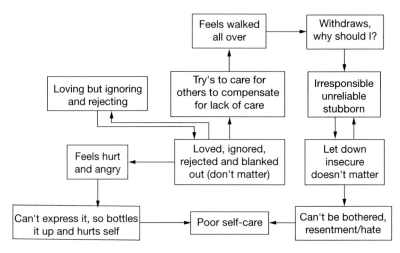

Figure 11.1 *CAT diagram for June – a self-destructive patient with unstable type 1 diabetes.*

So June's internalized parental roles revealed themselves in the therapy room. She expressed them, she elicited them and re-enacted them in relation to her self-care. Interpreting how blanking out/not mattering was continually re-enacted and made others reject her was very much the focus of June's therapy.

Countertransference

June invited me to blank her out when she did not respond or was stroppy; in particular, when she said, 'If you bother, why should I?' I wanted to resentfully ignore her! But this trap was interpreted and brought back to its roots so that the invitation was declined. We also spoke very little about June's actual diabetes, but we spoke about her feelings, her family and her social relationships. I was, however, feeling something that June was not, and that needed to be used in our work together. I felt some sort of hurt, which, given her history (and very much aided by the diagram), knew belonged to her, but she could not own – it was too painful. Thus, my feelings could be interpreted back to June as unexpressed versions of her own feelings which she could not herself access. This was also part of the work.

Responding to June's feelings began to stop her feeling blanked out. She began to feel vaguely important. This processed towards her thinking what it could be like to think that she mattered. And if she did matter, would this mean that she could provide herself with the antidote to her mother and father's care: i.e. that she could be reliable and responsible and elicit that care from others.

It was up to the therapy to model this antidote by providing good enough care that was to do with June being a loveable likeable human being. Her diagram made her feel as if she mattered ('that's me!'). Once she threw it at her parents as part of her initial attempts at not bottling things up: 'That's how I feel!' The re-enactments on the diagram were closely monitored throughout her therapy, so that June began to *recognize* connections and paradoxes between her own self-care and that received from her parents, and how she was repeating a pattern she 'hated'.

The aim of June's CAT was to improve her psychological well-being to the extent that she did not feel compelled to self-destruct. By the end of her therapy, she felt that she mattered. June transformed once she felt valued by significant others as a person apart from her illness. She began to be assertive and clear with others about her feelings and needs. This actually brought positive responses from others, including her parents. Six months after ending therapy June described how shocked she was to discover that she actually knew very little about her diabetes – her resistance had resulted in ignorance. She was seeing her specialist nurses *and* taking their advice! June's HbA_{1c} level, 3 months after this meeting, was 8.2%.

Conclusion

All patients referred to the psychotherapy service are neglectful or self-sabotaging in relation to their lives and their diabetes management. Their early formative experiences reveal that pre-diagnosis difficulties will later affect their diabetes management, so that diabetes gets 'caught up' in these early experiences. The causes and subsequent mechanisms of their difficulties are all different, and have been highlighted elsewhere.[18] The medical problem of diabetes and the emotional difficulties which interfere with management demonstrate the need for an individual approach to treatment which needs to address wide-ranging aspects of an individual's life as opposed to aiming for specific behavioural change in respect to detailed management techniques. CAT has been successful in the long term for these reasons, but also because the service occurs within the framework of the diabetes team. Patients are not sent outside the diabetes centre for psychological help; the psychological, metabolic and dietetic aspects of the patients are treated and discussed. Thus, the psychological in diabetes is acceptable, and part of the normal spectrum of diabetes care. Both patients and staff find this very helpful.

References

1. National Service Framework for Diabetes: Standards. Department of Health, 2002.
2. Lorenz RA, Bubb J, Davis D et al. Changing behavior: practical lessons from the Diabetes Control and Complications Trial. Diabetes Care 1996; 19: 648–52.
3. Snoek FJ, Skinner TC. Psychological counselling in problematic diabetes: does it help? Diabet Med 2002; 19: 265–73.
4. Rubin RR, Peyrot M. Psychosocial problems and interventions. A review of the literature. Diabetes Care 1992; 15: 1640–57.
5. Ryle A. Cognitive analytic therapy – active participation in change. John Wiley & Sons, Chichester, 1990.
6. Charman DP (ed.). Core processes in brief dynamic psychotherapy: training for effectiveness. New Jersey: Lawrence Erlbaum Associates, 2004.
7. Fosbury JA, Moore SM, Kidd JM, Sonksen PH, Amiel S. Psychological issues in the diabetes clinic. Pract Diabetes Intern 1996; 13: 92–3.
8. Milton J. Brief psychotherapy with poorly controlled diabetics. Br J Psychother 1989; 5: 532–43.
9. Fosbury JA, Bosley CM, Ryle A, Sonksen PH, Judd SL. A trial of cognitive analytic therapy in poorly controlled type 1 patients. Diabetes Care 1997; 20: 959–64.
10. Cowmeadow P. Deliberate self-harm and cognitive analytic therapy. Int J Short-term Psychother 1994; 9: 135–50.
11. Ryle A. Psychotherapy for grief and depression. Curr Opin Psychiatry 1991; 4: 371–4.

12. Walsh A, Hagan T, Gamsu D. Rescuer and rescued: applying a cognitive analytic perspective to explore the 'mis-management' of asthma. Br J Med Psychol 2002; 73: 151–68.
13. Ryle A. Cognitive analytic therapy and borderline personality disorder. The model and the method. John Wiley & Sons, Chichester, 1997.
14. Ryle A, Boa C, Fosbury JA. Identifying the causes of poor self management in insulin dependent diabetics. The use of cognitive analytic therapy techniques. In: Hodes M, Moorey S, eds. Psychological treatment in disease and illness. London: Gaskill, 1993.
15. Fosbury J. Psychological support for people with diabetes. A routine part of clinical care? Curr Med Lit Diabetes 1999; 16: 57–9.
16. Lockwood K. Integration in psychotherapy, is it possible? Paper presented by Dr Jane Milton. Association for Psychoanalytic Psychotherapy in the NHS. Newsletter 1991; 26: 4–5.
17. Fosbury JA. Psychological treatment (CAT) with poorly controlled type 1 patients. Pract Diabetes Int 1996; 13: 140–68.
18. Fosbury JA. The case study: the therapy, the patient and the therapist. In: Charman D, ed., Core processes in brief dynamic psychotherapy: training for effectiveness. New Jersey: Lawrence Erlbaum Associates, 2004.

chapter 12

Educational strategies for improving outcome in unstable diabetes

Helen Cooper

Introduction

Taken as a generic term, patient education covers a wide range of activities aimed at helping people to learn how to self-manage their disease. Essentially, it refers to a process of psycho-education, which the Delphi Group[1] has defined as:

> A planned learning experience using a combination of methods such as teaching, counselling, and behaviour modification techniques which influence patients' knowledge and health behaviour.

This definition acknowledges the importance of providing the patient with interventions that incorporate psycho-behavioural methods and psychosocial support, as well as the information and skills required to manage diabetes. While people with 'brittle diabetes' (the term used here to represent people with both brittle and unstable glycaemic control) represent a relatively small group of patients, they also demand a great deal of professional time, with frequent hospital admissions representing one of the defining features.[2] This suggests that education has minimal impact. Such a pattern implies that there is a need to go back to the drawing board and review the mechanisms that underlie such activities. These mechanisms relate to theoretical frameworks, teaching strategies and evaluation strategies.

Theoretical frameworks

Theories of adult education

Theories associated with adult education can be traced back to the work of various educational theorists who identified five domains of learning in which change may take place: knowledge, skills, understanding, attitudes and application. These domains were developed from psychological theories which, for convenience, can be divided into three main groups: cognitive, behaviourist and humanist theories and are briefly discussed next.

Cognitive theories of learning

Cognitive theories are concerned with how knowledge is acquired and point to the active engagement of the mind in relation to the matter under consideration. Cognitive psychologists believe that learning is an internal process concerned with thinking, perception, organization and insight. Brewin[3] considers that the cognitive nature of learning demands that individuals understand what has been happening to them, what has been learned from it and what the consequences are thought to be for the future. Meaningful learning is thus achieved through a process of reflection. This suggests the need for the teacher to provide a scaffolding of ideas to bridge the gap between what the patient already knows to what he needs to know before he can learn the new material in a meaningful fashion. This approach is appropriate for adult learners who have a lot of previous knowledge and experiences and are able to manipulate ideas. Education should therefore be related to what has gone on before in the patient's life.

Behaviourist theories of learning

According to behaviourists, most behaviour is learned by making a link or connection between a stimulus and a response. The process by which a link is made is called conditioning. There are three types of conditioning: classical, operant and vicarious. Pavlov (1849–1936) is perhaps the best known for his work on classical conditioning when he linked one stimulus, meat powder, to a second stimulus, a bell sound, to produce a response of salivation in dogs. After conditioning, the dogs would salivate to the sound of a bell (conditioned stimulus), even in the absence of the meat powder (unconditioned stimulus). Pavlov found that once a response had been conditioned, it could then be produced by other stimuli similar to the conditioned response, a process he called generalization. Such classical conditioning has been found to have value in understanding the learning of emotional responses to certain situations. It has been used in education and counselling to extinguish already established fear/anxiety responses and to establish the role of providing learners with cues prior to a behaviour being performed to remind them of the expected behaviour.

Operant conditioning, or trial-and-error learning, works on the principle that humans behave in such a way as to receive gratification. The behaviour (response) occurs first and is followed by a consequence that gives satisfaction and so becomes a stimulus. The theory of operant conditioning can be credited to the work of Thorndike (1874–1949) and Skinner (1904–90). Thorndike proposed that behaviour which results in success is more likely to be repeated than behaviour which does not. He also suggested that repetition of successful actions results in considerable learning and this achievement is enjoyable for the learner. Skinner emphasized the use of reinforcement as the key to learning. Positive reinforcement is used to encourage a behaviour, while negative reinforcement (or absence of reinforcement) is used to extinguish the non-desirable behaviour. Operant conditioning has been widely applied in clinical settings (i.e. for behaviour modification) as well as teaching (i.e. for classroom management). Kemm and Close[4] describe how it is used in health promotion, where activities that are planned to be relevant to the needs of clients, are interesting and are within the client's capabilities are more likely to be successful.

The theories associated with vicarious conditioning were developed by Bandura,[5] who developed the theory of social learning. Vicarious conditioning involves the observed behaviour of others and the consequences of those behaviours. If the consequences are perceived to be desirable, the behaviour may be copied or modelled. If the consequences are seen to be undesirable, the behaviour may be avoided. Hence, learning can occur vicariously through the behaviour of others (modelling). Vicarious conditioning relates to the notion of 'reciprocal determinism' and to the concept of self-efficacy. Reciprocal determinism, whereby an individual learns continuously to assess his or her interaction with society and the environment and subconsciously to accept behavioural influence (social norms), is central to health promotion practice. Bandura further developed this idea through the notion of self-efficacy, which he defined as the 'belief in one's capabilities to organise and execute the sources of action required to manage prospective situations'.[6] This proposes that individuals will undertake certain behaviour changes only if there is a belief in them being successful. Self-efficacy is considered to be the single most important aspect of learners' efforts to change their behaviour because it removes doubts about their abilities to modify current patterns of behaviour. It influences personal choice, the amount of effort and persistence put into changing behaviour and the ability to confront obstacles to change.

Humanist theories of learning

Humanist theories of learning are concerned with feelings and experiences leading to personal growth and individual fulfilment. Maslow[7] made a significant contribution to the humanist approach with his theory of motivation and hierarchy of needs. Maslow claimed that there is a hierarchy of human needs, and basic physical needs must be satisfied before the higher cognitive needs can be achieved. His general theory was that the function of education is ultimately the 'self-actualization' of a person, or what he described as the process of helping people to become the best that they are able to become. To achieve this goal he stressed the need to understand the psychology of the learner to provide a base for the 'understanding of what a person can communicate to the world and what the world is able to communicate to him'.

In relation to patient education, humanist theories highlight the importance of facilitating understanding of the emotional aspects of learning to live with a chronic disease before higher cognitive needs can be achieved. Lazarus[8] argued that to help people cope better with the stress of an illness they need to be aware of what they are coping with. Hernandez[9] researched experiences of living with diabetes and found that as the emotional impact of the disease lessened so the ability to self-manage the disease improved.

Comparison of the three theories

The three groups of theories described are complementary. They stress that:

- learning is achieved by making new information meaningful to the learner by linking it to that already known (cognitive theories)
- behaviour is influenced by the meaning attached to it and the perceived consequences (behaviourist theories)
- feelings and experiences need to be acknowledged before higher cognitive needs can be achieved (humanist theories).

These three principles acknowledge that adults learn best when their learning relates to life experiences. Such an approach describes experiential learning which is associated with various educational philosophers, including Dewey, Kolb, Knowles, Brookfield, Jarvis and Rogers. They have proposed certain principles for facilitating adult learning which been translated into teaching strategies.

Teaching strategies

Experiential learning

The work of Dewey[10] best articulates the guiding principles for programmes of adult experiential learning. As long ago as 1952, he argued that there is an intimate and necessary relation between the processes of actual experience and education. He believed that the knowledge, skills and social experiences that people bring with them to education have value for others, including the teacher, whose role is to decide which experiences are educative. As Dewey wrote, 'the central problem of an education based upon experience is to select the kind of present experiences that live fruitfully and creatively in subsequent experiences'. Dewey was at the forefront of a movement away from the traditional methods of teaching.

The learning cycle

Kolb[11] devised the 'learning cycle', which he linked to the work of Dewey and also to the work of Lewin (1890–1947) and Piaget (1896–1980). Lewin's theories emphasize learning as a dialectic process that integrates experience and concepts, observations, and actions. Piaget's cognitive theory defines the developmental processes from birth that shape the basic learning processes of adults. Kolb's learning cycle includes four stages of experiential learning: concrete experience, reflective observation, abstract conceptualization and active experimentation. This model defines learning as a continuous process grounded in experience, so that the emphasis is on the process of adaptation and learning, as opposed to content or outcomes. A hallmark of the experiential learning theory is its acknowledgement of the human side of learning, taking into account the role of emotional feelings and choice, alongside cognition.

Adragogy versus pedagogy

Knowles[12] used the term 'adragogy' to describe the process of adult experiential learning in order to distinguish it from the principles that guide the teaching of children (pedagogy). He described four main assumptions of adragogy that are different from those of pedagogy. Brookfield[13] also independently proposed certain principles for facilitating adult learning which concurred with those of Knowles:

- Adults both desire and enact a tendency toward self-directedness as they mature, though they may be dependent in certain circumstances.
- Adults' experiences are a rich resource for learning. Adults learn more effectively through experiential techniques of education such as discussion or problem solving.
- Adults are aware of specific learning needs generated by real-life tasks or problems. Adult education programmes should therefore be organized around 'life application' categories and sequenced according to learners' readiness to learn.
- Adults are competency-based learners in that they wish to apply newly acquired skills or knowledge to their immediate circumstances. Adults are therefore 'performance-centred' in their orientation to learning.[14]

Attributes of the teacher

Jarvis[15] described adult education as an interactive process because a relationship is necessarily formed between the 'teacher' and the 'learner'. He argued that because education involves human relationships, it is essentially a moral interaction. This argument supports the work of Rogers,[16] who identified three basic moral attributes of the teacher:

- integrity – being genuine, trustworthy and honest with learners and with ones self
- respect – showing kindness and caring for the welfare of learners and recognizing their individual autonomy and differences
- compassion – empathizing with the learner, helping him/her to recognize and deal with important issues which may involve sharing individual emotional responses to shared experiences.

These attributes are especially important when dealing with patients who have unstable diabetes, which may be indicative of an unresolved grieving process associated with the diagnosis of diabetes, and perhaps with other stressful experiences in their lives. Next to the death of a loved one, the diagnosis of a chronic disease is one of the more stressful events facing adults and leaves way for a profound experience of loss and emotional disruption. Helping patients understand their reactions should be an integral part of the educational process so that diabetes can eventually be internalized to form a fundamental part of their self-concept. Without such intervention, a vicious cycle of helplessness accompanied by feelings of powerlessness and passive dependence may ensue. This can lead to either an outward expression of anger, destructive activities and associated guilt feelings or to anger directed inwardly (denial), resulting in symptoms of depression. Both reactions operate on an unconscious level and perpetuation impairs an individual's ability to cope with everyday problems of living.[17] Patient education is therefore directed at interrupting this cycle to promote resolution of the loss. It highlights that learning to live with diabetes is a transformation process that is being continuously created and recreated. As such, it is not an independent entity to be transferred didactically by the teacher. Such cognitive learning recognizes a humanistic approach to education that acknowledges the importance of understanding the characteristics of patients and their individual needs so that interventions can be tailored accordingly.

Learner characteristics

As long ago as 1963, Houle[18] stressed that to understand education we must begin by understanding the nature, the beliefs and the actions of those taking part, which can provide useful insights and understanding of learners' needs. Without this understanding, educational interventions will probably achieve objectives other than those that have been planned. Houle's work demonstrated that the real worth and meaning of any educational activity resides with the learner, rather than with the teacher. From this perspective, the role of health professionals is to obtain a detailed assessment of patients' characteristics and their learning needs so that educational plans can be designed accordingly. Such an assessment calls for an evaluation strategy to explore the reasons behind failures to adopt recommended health protective behaviours. This requires understanding of the theoretical processes by which such behaviours are acquired.

Evaluation strategies

All patients with diabetes face several unique behavioural challenges which they are encouraged to comply with to prevent complications. Croyle and Ditto[19] relate such health protective behaviour to 'any mental activity (e.g. appraisal, interpretation, recall) undertaken by an individual who believes himself or herself to be ill, regarding the state of his or her health and its possible remedies'. This definition stresses the need for educational interventions to be aligned to patients' needs, so that they can develop positive coping strategies.

The challenges of living with diabetes: developing coping mechanisms

There has been growing interest in the cognitive and behavioural strategies patients use to manage diabetes, reflecting recognition of the importance of individual coping mechanisms. Various factors have been proposed, including, for example, attitudes, threat appraisals and emotional responses. These variables link into a variety of theoretical perspectives, including:

- process-orientated models, in particular personal models of illness
- expectancy value models, e.g. health belief model, health locus of control, theory of planned behaviour, transtheoretical stages-of-change model.

Deciding which of these theoretical perspectives is relevant is less important than deciding which variables and processes within these theories can improve our understanding of patient education. Although it is beyond this chapter to consider all the theories in detail, two models are worth describing, as they have particular relevance to patients with brittle diabetes. These are the personal models of illness and the transtheoretical stages-of-change model.

Personal models of illness

Illness representations fit closely with a concept of illness behaviour as a response to the problematic experience of illness, including consideration of the way people respond to the diagnosis of an illness. Recent research has focused on identification of the way in which individuals organize and process information about their illness, i.e. peoples' mental representations of their disease. This includes their emotions, knowledge, experiences and beliefs about their disease. This field of psychological research has been well served by Leventhal.[20-22] His work has shown how patients evaluate health threats by constructing their own personal models of their illness, which influence their patterns of coping. He has found that these so-called 'common-sense models of illness' are derived in part from the social environment and from past illness experiences. He identified four attributes of individuals' representations of illness threats:

1. identity (disease label and associated knowledge)
2. consequences (short or long term)
3. time-line (temporal course)
4. attributes concerning the cause of the problem.[19]

A fifth component was subsequently added – cure (for acute diseases) or controllability (for chronic diseases). Leventhal et al[20] proposed that these representations, which are not necessarily independent, are processed in parallel to patients' emotional responses to the illness.

A team of researchers have investigated personal model constructs in relation to diabetes.[23-26] Through their work, they have demonstrated that three explicit aspects of illness representations are predictive of certain diabetes self-management activities. These are:

- *Treatment effectiveness* – perceived helpfulness of treatment, including self-care and satisfaction with care
- *Seriousness* – beliefs about current seriousness, impact on lifestyle and emotions, and likelihood of and worry about future complications

■ *Personal control* – including beliefs about degree of personal responsibility in the past for 'causing' their diabetes.

Hampson et al[27] highlight how these constructs have been found to be predictive of both current and prospective self-care activities, with the most predictive of the constructs being treatment effectiveness. This is similar to the concept of self-efficacy, because both assess beliefs about the link between actions and outcomes and relate to personal choice and to the amount of effort and persistence put into self-care.

Personal model representations come into play as soon as patients experience their initial symptoms and typically change with disease progression, emergent symptoms and treatment responses. They therefore represent a dynamic process which can change according to personal experiences. This has particular relevance to patients with brittle diabetes. It highlights how perceptions of the need for change are intricately linked with past experiences and what patients believe to be of importance to them. It also acknowledges the relevance of patients' emotional responses to their disease, which are a significant aspect of their experiences of illness. Helping patients to reassess their personal models of diabetes may therefore allow learning to become more meaningful

Transtheoretical stages-of-change model

This model is derived from the work of Prochaska and DiClemente,[28–30] who worked with a variety of addictive behaviours (e.g. smoking, alcohol use, compulsive eating), as well as health protective behaviours (e.g. weight control and physical exercise). Their work has shown that behaviour change involves an intrinsic process that alters the way clients view the necessary changes expected of them. Aveyard et al[29] highlight how this process includes decisional balance factors (the balance of the pros and cons of a particular behaviour), self-efficacy and temptations to relapse. This approach removes the belief that behaviour change is an all or nothing approach. Five stages in the transtheoretical model of change have been described by Prochaska et al,[30] and these are summarized in Table 12.1.

Table 12.1 The five stages of behaviour change

Stage	Description
Precontemplation – not interested in changing behaviour	Do not know that current behaviour is risky or fully aware of risks but value current behaviour and do not wish to change
Contemplation – considering change in the foreseeable future but no commitment to change	Raised awareness about risks of behaviour but ambivalent about change. Balance will shift either way for reasons that are unique to each individual
Preparation – intention to change in the near future	Beginning to make clear plans on how to carry out chosen behaviour change(s)
Action – in the process of changing behaviour	Often engage with health professionals or self-help groups or engage in self-change strategies at this stage
Maintenance – continued change for an extended period with emphasis on preventing relapse	Change in behaviour continued and consolidated. Temporary change becomes a more settled pattern. At this stage, termination or permanent maintenance may be achieved
Relapse – return to one of the other stages	An integral part of the change process. May occur at any stage and therefore does not mean the end of the process

Whereas many of the variables in the model can also be found in other theories of health protective behaviours, Prochaska et al[30] have focused attention on behaviour change as a spiral (as opposed to a linear) process. This assumes that the adoption of healthy behaviours involves a series of decisions and consists of several stages which patients move through in either direction (progress or relapse). Such an approach is important because it recognizes that several attempts at change may be appropriate in order to learn and practice a new behaviour before eventually achieving a goal of maintenance of the behaviour. The spiral pattern indicates that most people learn from their relapse experiences rather than going in circles without any progress at all. From this perspective, success is identified as a client's progress toward change, rather than waiting for the outcome to be realized.

This model has particular relevance for people with brittle diabetes. It suggests that they may, for example, be in the 'precontemplation' phase of change – not recognizing that their behaviours are risky, or else they value their current behaviour and do not wish to change it. It may be that they are receiving reinforcement for their maladaptive behaviours (frequent hospitalizations and associated attention, for example) which encourages continuance of the behaviour. This provides foci for intervention. For example, assessing patients' perceptions of the importance of the recommended behaviour change and the level of confidence they have to take such change forward can provide guidelines for intervention. Figure 12.1 outlines various strategies that can be implemented at each of the stages of the cycle of change and shows that attitude change is a prerequisite to behaviour change. It also shows how they link into the theories underpinning patient education, with their focus on experiential learning, patients' characteristics and emotional adaptation.

Bringing the theories together

It can be seen that there are variables common to all the theories described. This suggests that the number of truly distinct factors

**Permanent
maintenance
or termination**

⇧

Success!
Well done
Review process with client

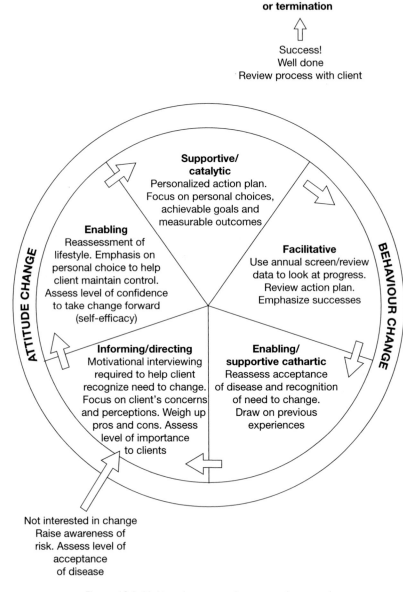

**Supportive/
catalytic**
Personalized action plan.
Focus on personal choices,
achievable goals and
measurable outcomes

Enabling
Reassessment of
lifestyle. Emphasis on
personal choice to help
client maintain control.
Assess level of confidence
to take change forward
(self-efficacy)

Facilitative
Use annual screen/review
data to look at progress.
Review action plan.
Emphasize successes

ATTITUDE CHANGE

BEHAVIOUR CHANGE

Informing/directing
Motivational interviewing
required to help client
recognize need to change.
Focus on client's concerns
and perceptions. Weigh up
pros and cons. Assess
level of importance
to clients

**Enabling/
supportive cathartic**
Reassess acceptance
of disease and recognition
of need to change.
Draw on previous
experiences

Not interested in change
Raise awareness of
risk. Assess level of
acceptance
of disease

Figure 12.1 *Making changes: a client-centred approach.*

relevant to patient education is considerably lower than might have been expected. These factors include:

1. cognitive factors, i.e. attitudes and self-related beliefs, including perceptions of self-efficacy
2. social–environmental variables, e.g. social norms, influences of friends, family, health care providers
3. psychological factors, i.e. perceptions of treatment effectiveness, seriousness and personal control, including emotional reactions to the disease.

Whereas the concept of empowering patients to take control of their disease is considered to be central to all patient education activities, the synergistic relationship between these variables needs to be considered. This highlights the dynamic nature of patient education which needs to work on affecting change in all the factors noted. Such a spectrum of variables is encompassed in Tones and Tilford's[31] definition of health education, which appropriately amalgamates the theoretical and practical constructs associated with this activity:

> Health education is any intentional activity which is designed
> to achieve health or illness related learning, i.e. some
> relatively permanent change in an individual's capability or
> disposition. Effective health education may thus produce
> changes in knowledge and understanding on ways of
> thinking; it may influence or clarify values; it may bring about
> some shift in belief or attitude; it may facilitate the acquisition
> of skills; it may even effect changes in behaviour or lifestyle.

This definition suggests that education is a long-term process that needs to follow a detailed scheme which is written into an integrated care plan to ensure consistency between the interprofessional team. The theories described so far provide the framework for such intervention as they can be used to direct assessment, intervention and evaluation.

Table 12.2 Brief comparative summary of the theories, teaching strategies and evaluation techniques associated with patient education

	Cognitive	Behaviourist	Humanist
Theoretical framework	*Knowledge/skills*: Link prior knowledge/experiences with new information *Attitudes*: Formulate new ideas through process of deduction *Understanding*: Insightful learning gained through adaptation of existing knowledge or past experiences to form new insights	Behaviour learnt by making a link between a stimulus and a response (conditioned responses) Development of self-efficacy, which removes doubts about abilities to modify behaviour Learning achieved through repetition of successful actions (trial-and-error learning, operant conditioning, copying others' behaviours, vicarious conditioning)	Higher cognitive needs to be met by understanding the psychological factors influencing behaviour Development of awareness and understanding of attitudes toward certain situations Insightful learning gained through understanding personal feelings to certain situations
Teaching strategies: *Application for learner*	Learning seen as a process of thinking, perception, organization and insight. Associated with problem-solving approaches to learning	Development of understanding of how emotional responses are related to certain situations. Associated with education and counselling to extinguish established fear/anxiety responses and behaviour modification	Confrontation of personal problems to gain insight into emotional responses. Associated with patient education to facilitate understanding of the emotional aspects of learning to live with a chronic disease

Application for teacher	Need to make new information meaningful to learners by linking it to that already known	Need to use reinforcement – positively to reinforce behaviour, negatively to prevent repetition of behaviour. Behaviour of teacher provides a model for learners to copy (see opposite)	Need to show integrity, respect and compassion toward learners
Evaluation techniques	Look for changes in: • knowledge, skills and understanding (insight) • ability to identify problem areas, i.e. discrepancy between current status and desired goals	Look for: • changes in risk awareness and ambivalence • personalized action planning for behaviour change (personal goals) • behaviour change – permanent maintenance or relapse – as an integral part of behaviour change spiral	Look for changes in: • relationship with 'teacher' – move toward collaborative working • mutual problem-solving • attitudes toward diabetes and its treatment • personal models of diabetes

Adapted from Cooper H, Booth K, Gill G. Patients' perspectives on diabetes health care education. Health Education Research 2003; 18(2): 191–206, by permission of Oxford University Press.

Practice implications

Taking theory as the framework for psycho-education, the next question is what competencies are required to manage the educational process. Research with patients who have type 2 diabetes highlighted the following attributes they valued:[32–35]

- protected time for health professionals to devote to teaching
- expertise, empathy and personal commitment to the educational process
- learner-centred approach
- augmentation of prior knowledge so that new information and experiences are integrated with existing knowledge and experiences
- use of reflection to provide time for reappraisal to clarify and interpret the complexities of diabetes self-management
- collaborative approach to learning between patient and health professional, with personal experience likened to expertise
- supportive environment created by a group approach to learning
- increased motivation by learning from peers and shared empathy for difficulties encountered when living with diabetes in the 'real world'.

Patients clearly demonstrate that psychological changes are as much a primary focus of educational intervention as providing the knowledge and skills for self-care. Although entry into the behaviour change cycle is the primary aim of intervention, progress is reliant upon continued support from family, friends, health professionals, etc. Termination of change can only be achieved when diabetes becomes an integral part of patients' lives and not an external matter to be taken care of before they get on with the business of living. In effect, this reflects a process of integration of the personal and the diabetic selves so that they become unified.[9]

Conclusions

The original aim of this chapter was to review the mechanisms that underlie patient education: namely theoretical frameworks, teaching strategies and evaluation strategies. Critical to the success of patient education is an understanding of how these mechanisms relate to each other. Table 12.2 provides a descriptive summary of this relationship. It demonstrates that ongoing needs assessment and evaluation is a vital ingredient of educational planning and that such a process must be an integral part of patient care. In this way interventions can be targeted according to evolving needs. The role of the teacher (in this case the health professional), then becomes one of a mentor to patients so that they can be supported and guided through their diabetes journey. Such mentorship is obviously more likely to be successful when the teacher has a good understanding of the mechanisms underlying patient education. This takes us back to the very beginning of the chapter. It shows that questions come before answers, and that a teacher's job is never finished.

References

1. Delphi Group. Patient education terminology. Patient Education and Counseling 1985; 7: 323–4.
2. Gill GV. Does brittle diabetes exist? In: Gill G, Pickup JC, Williams G, eds, Difficult diabetes. Blackwell Science, Oxford, 2001, pp 151–68.
3. Brewin CR. Cognitive foundations of clinical psychology. Lawrence Erlbaum Associates, London, 1988.
4. Kemm J, Close A (Eds). Health promotion, theory and practice. Macmillan Press, London, 1995.
5. Bandura A. Self-efficacy: towards a unifying theory of behavioral change. Psycholog Rev 1977; 84: 191–215.
6. Bandura A. Self-efficacy mechanism in human agency. Am Psychol 1982; 37: 122–47.
7. Maslow AH. The farther reaches of human nature. The Viking Press, New York, 1971.
8. Lazarus RS. Coping with the stress of illness. In: Kaplun A, ed, Health promotion and chronic illness: discovering a new quality of health. WHO

published in association with the Federal Centre of Health Education, Copenhagen, 1974, pp 11–31.

9. Hernandez CA. Integration: the experience of living with insulin dependent (Type 1) diabetes mellitus. Can J Nurs Res 1996; 28: 37–56.
10. Dewey J. Education and experience. The Macmillan Company, New York, 1952.
11. Kolb DA. Experiential learning: experience as the source of learning and development. Prentice Hall, Englewood Cliffs, New Jersey, 1984.
12. Knowles MS. The adult learner: a neglected species. Gulf Publishing Company, Houston, Texas, 1973.
13. Brookfield SD. Understanding and facilitating adult learning. Open University Press, Milton Keynes, 1986.
14. Knowles MS and Associates. Adragogy in action: applying modern principles of adult learning. Jossey-Bass, San Francisco, 1984.
15. Jarvis P. Teachers and learners in adult education: transaction or moral interaction?. Stud Educ Adults 1995; 27: 24–35.
16. Rogers A. Teaching adults. Open University Press, Milton Keynes, 1986.
17. Drake RE, Price JL. Depression: adaptation to disruption and loss. Psychiatric Care 1975; XIII: 163–9.
18. Houle CO. The inquiring mind. The University of Wisconsin Press, Madison, 1963.
19. Croyle RT, Ditto PH. Illness cognition and behaviour: an experimental approach. J Behav Med 1990; 13: 31–52.
20. Leventhal H, Meyer D, Nerenz D. The common sense representation of illness danger. In: Rachman S, ed., Contributions to medical psychology. Pergamon Press, Oxford, 1980, pp 7–30.
21. Leventhal H, Nerenz DR, Steele DJ. Illness representations and coping with health threats. In: Baum A, Taylor SE, Singer JE, eds, Handbook of psychology and health. Erlbaum, Hillside, New Jersey, 1984.
22. Leventhal H. Symptom reporting: a focus on process. In: McHugh S, Vallis TM, eds, Illness behaviour: a multidisciplinary model. Plenum Press, New York, 1986, pp 219–236.
23. Hampson S, Glasgow RE, Foster LS. Personal models of diabetes among older adults: relationships to self-management and other variables. The Diabetes Educator 1995; 21: 300–7.
24. Hampson HE, Glasgow RE, Stryker LA, Ruggiero L. Personal-model beliefs and socio-environmental barriers related to diabetes self-management. Diabetes Care 1997; 20: 556–61.
25. Skinner TC, Hampson SE. Personal models of diabetes in relation to self-care, well-being and glycemic control. Diabetes Care 2001; 24: 828–33.
26. Skinner TC, Hampson SE, Fife-Schaw C. Personality, personal model beliefs, and self-care in adolescents and young adults with Type 1 diabetes. Health Psychol 2002; 21: 61–70.
27. Hampson HE, Glasgow RE, Toobert DJ. Personal models of diabetes and their relations to self-care activities. Health Psychol 1990; 9: 632–46.

28. Prochaska JO, DiClemente CC. Stages and processes of self-change of smoking: toward an integrative model of change. J Consult Clin Psychol 1983; 51: 390–5.
29. Aveyard P, Cheng KK, Almond J et al. Cluster randomised controlled trial of expert system based on the transtheoretical ('stages of change') model for smoking prevention and cessation in schools. Br Med J 1999; 319: 948–53.
30. Prochaska JO, DiClemente CC, Norcross JC. In search of how people change: applications to addictive behaviours. Am Psychologist 1992; 47: 1102–14.
31. Tones K, Tilford S. Health education. Effectiveness, efficiency and equity. Chapman and Hall, London, 1994.
32. Cooper H. Capturing the impact of patient education for people with Type 2 diabetes. Unpublished PhD thesis, Liverpool University, 2001.
33. Cooper H, Booth K, Gill G. Diabetes education: the patient's perspective. J Diabet Nurs 2002; 6: 91–5.
34. Cooper H, Booth K, Gill G. Patients' perspectives on diabetes health care education. Health Education Research 2003; 18: 191–206.
35. Cooper H, Booth K, Gill G. Using combined research methods for exploring diabetes patient education. Patient Education and Counselling 2003; 51: 45–52.

chapter 13

Insulin pumps and pancreas transplantation for unstable and brittle diabetes

John Pickup

There has been a resurgence of interest in insulin infusion pump treatment for managing difficult diabetes in recent years and this has mostly centred on the use of continuous subcutaneous insulin infusion (CSII) in type 1 diabetic patients with frequent unpredictable hypoglycaemia. Indeed, the realization that CSII is so effective for this clinical problem has been one of the main stimuli for the increasing use of CSII in several countries.[1] Interestingly, the indications for CSII are similar to those of islet cell transplantation, where there has been new hope since the introduction of the novel Edmonton protocol in 2000.[2]

Table 13.1 Clinical problems in diabetes where CSII has been evaluated. Evidence that CSII is superior to multiple insulin injection therapy

A. Evidence for a substantial beneficial effect in type 1 diabetes
Frequent, unpredictable hypoglycaemia
Hypoglycaemia unawareness
Wide, unpredictable swings in glycaemia
Gastroparesis with associated hypoglycaemia
Poor control (hypoglycaemia, glycaemic oscillations) during diabetic pregnancy
Dawn phenomenon

B. No effect, or limited benefit in some type 1 diabetic subjects
Recurrent ketoacidosis/insulin resistance

C. Inconclusive evidence of effect
Poor control in type 2 diabetes

This chapter will focus on a number of clinical problems which constitute difficult or brittle diabetes and where pump therapy may be helpful; most experience has been with CSII (Table 13.1). More practical and technical details of pump therapy can be found elswhere.[3,4] Although little is yet known about islet and pancreas transplantation as a routine clinical treatment for unstable diabetes, a brief note on the potential for transplantation concludes the chapter.

Insulin infusion pumps

Hypoglycaemia
Troublesome hypoglycaemia in type 1 diabetes is the best-established indication for the use of CSII and is the clinical problem where

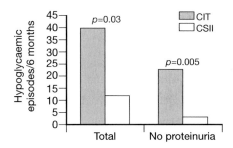

Figure 13.1 *Number of episodes of severe hypoglycaemia in a 6-month period in 40 type I diabetic patients treated by conventional insulin therapy (CIT) compared with a matched group of 40 type I patients treated by continuous subcutaneous insulin infusion (CSII). Total = all patients; no proteinuria = those without clinical (dipstick positive) proteinuria. (Data from reference 8.)*

evidence of benefit is most convincing.[1] Interestingly, in early uncontrolled anecdotal reports, hypoglycaemia was regarded as an adverse complication of pump therapy,[5,6] but numerous studies have now shown that a high frequency of severe or moderate hypoglycaemia during insulin injection therapy is markedly reduced during CSII.[7–11]

In an audit of CSII in the 1980s, it was observed that the frequency of hypoglycaemic coma was about one-third of that in injection-treated type 1 diabetic subjects of similar age, sex and duration of diabetes[8] (Fig. 13.1). A randomized controlled trial at about the same time (the Oslo Study) showed that severe hypoglycaemia was reduced by 85% during CSII, compared to multiple injection therapy. Most subsequent studies have compared hypoglycaemia in patients switched from multiple injections to pumps. A recent influential example is that of Bode et al,[9] where the incidence of severe hypoglycaemia in 55 type 1 diabetic patients was reduced from 138 during one year on multiple injections to 22 events per 100 patient-years in the first year of CSII, although glycated haemoglobin (HbA_{1c}) remained unchanged (Fig. 13.2). In another trial, 55 adolescents with type 1 diabetes who changed to CSII after 1 year on multiple injections had the frequency of severe hypoglycaemia reduced by nearly 50%, although the HbA_{1c} was significantly lower on pumps (7.5 vs

273

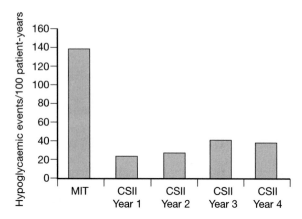

Figure 13.2 *Reduction in the frequency of severe hypoglycaemia in type 1 diabetic patients switched from multiple injection therapy (MIT) to continuous subcutaneous insulin infusion (CSII). (Data from Bode et al.[9])*

8.3%). A retrospective review of French patients being treated by CSII confirmed the beneficial effects of pumps on hypoglycaemia, finding a halving in the number of patients with ≥1 severe event per year and an overall reduction of 77% in the number of events per year.[11]

Lesser degrees of hypoglycaemia may also be improved by CSII. A recent meta-analysis of randomized controlled trials[12] showed that the overall glycaemic control in type 1 diabetic patients not selected for control problems is only slightly better during CSII than on multiple injections (about 1 mmol/l lower for the mean blood glucose concentration and 0.5% for HbA_{1c}), but oscillations in blood glucose are reduced by some 20% (Fig. 13.3), perhaps reflecting the lower variability of subcutaneous insulin absorption from pumps compared to injection therapy.[13] Unpredictable oscillations in blood glucose short of severe hypoglycaemia represent a debilitating pattern of poor control in some diabetic patients, which can worsen to multiple hypoglycaemic events when attempts are made to tighten control. The well-being and quality of life of such patients can often be markedly improved by CSII, although there is often little change in the crude index of HbA_{1c} percentage.

Recurrent hypoglycaemia is a major factor in the pathogenesis of hypoglycaemia unawareness[14,15] and several studies have demon-

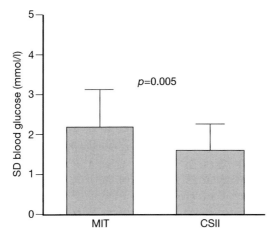

Figure 13.3 *Reduction in the variability of blood glucose concentrations during continuous subcutaneous insulin infusion (CSII) compared to multiple injection therapy (MIT), as assessed by the standard deviation (SD) of daily blood glucose values. Data are from a meta-analysis of 12 randomized controlled trials comparing glycaemic control during CSII and MIT.*[12]

strated that rigorous avoidance of hypoglycaemia restores hypogly-caemia awareness to a greater or lesser extent.[16–18] In this respect, the relatively simple strategy of changing the night-time isophane insulin injection to night-time CSII at the basal rate was found to improve warning symptoms, decrease the variability of the fasting glucose level and to reduce the frequency of blood glucose values <3.5 mmol/l.[19]

A number of case reports have described patients with long-stand-ing type 1 diabetes complicated by gastroparesis, frequent hypo-glycaemia and hypoglycaemia unawareness during optimized insulin injection treatment, where the frequency of hypoglycaemia has been improved by CSII.[20,21] Although autonomic neuropathy itself may not be significantly altered by improved glycaemic control,[22] disordered gastric emptying may be independent of neuropathy and normogly-caemia may improve gastroparesis.[23] Modern insulin pumps have the facility for an extended square-wave prandial bolus delivery, which may help in the management of such patients with gastroparesis.

Recurrent ketoacidosis and insulin resistance

Continuous subcutaneous insulin infusion

Recurrent diabetic ketoacidosis (DKA) is a relatively rare problem in type 1 diabetes, often affecting young females.[24-26] Many are apparently receiving large doses of insulin by subcutaneous injection, a mean of about 7 units/kg vs 1.0 unit/kg in matched non-brittle females,[24] and are regarded by many as the classical 'brittle' diabetic patient. We[24,27] and others[28,29] have reported that glycaemic control is not usually improved by CSII in these patients (Fig. 13.4). In a series of 12 female brittle diabetic patients studied at our centre the mean plasma glucose concentration during CSII varied from 9.8 to 19.1 mmol/l with continued wide swings in blood glucose, and a standard deviation of values ranging from 4.0 (range 3.4–20.1) to 12.3 (range 1.1–45) mmol/l in individual patients. In 30 type 1 diabetic patients with incapacitating brittle diabetes described by Schade et al,[28] 70% had unsuccessfully tried CSII.

There are a few reported cases of diabetic patients with recurrent DKA who have benefited from CSII, with reduced hospital admissions and lower but not nearly normalized HbA$_{1c}$ percentages. Steindel et

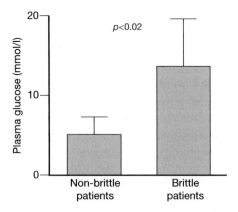

Figure 13.4 *Glycaemic control during continuous subcutaneous insulin infusion (CSII) in 5 non-brittle type 1 diabetic patients compared with 5 brittle diabetic patients characterized by recurrent ketoacidosis. (Data from Pickup et al.[27])*

al[30] described 6 children aged 8–16 years who had had at least 2 episodes of DKA per year for up to 7 years. Four of the patients were thought to be non-adherent to their prescribed insulin injection therapy. When switched to CSII, there was a 50% reduction in DKA and a 75% reduction in the number of days in hospital at 1 year. HbA$_{1c}$ remained the same at 9%. Also, Blackett[31] reported on 4 adolescent girls with type 1 diabetes and multiple admissions to hospital with DKA, where CSII achieved a reduction in hospitalization, although no significant change in HbA$_{1c}$ at 1 year.

Perhaps some young patients are more compliant with a simple CSII regimen than with multiple injections. A basal infusion may afford sufficient insulinization to avoid many potential episodes of DKA, even when meal boluses are forgotten. This is in accord with the study of Nathan,[29] where, reasoning that erratic absorption of meal boluses was the source of difficult diabetic control, a variable basal rate infusion that omitted boluses was employed. Generally, a high basal rate (2–6 units/h) was employed from about 8 a.m. to 9 a.m., with two reduced rates (daytime and nightime) thereafter. The frequency of DKA and hypoglycaemia was reduced with this infusion regimen. In these studies of the 'successful' use of CSII in recurrent DKA, virtually no patient was free of ketoacidosis on insulin pump therapy, with, for example, a mean of 1.7 episodes per patient-year during CSII in the study of Steindel et al.[30] This is far higher than the rates of 0.02–0.07 episodes/patient-year reported in non-brittle type diabetic subjects treated by CSII.[8–10,32]

Another report refers to an older subject suffering from repeated hypoglycaemic and hyperglycaemic coma during injection therapy, 51 years old at the time of starting CSII, who was successfully treated by pump therapy for 20 years.[33] The underlying cause of the instability was hypoadrenalism and hypothyroidism.

Continuous intravenous insulin infusion

It has often been surmised that poor control in brittle or insulin-resistant diabetic subjects is due to a subcutaneous barrier to insulin absorption,[27] and several groups have therefore attempted to improve control in such patients by continuous intravenous insulin infusion (CIVII) from a portable pump. Dandona et al[34] were one of the first to employ this strategy, reporting on 6 diabetic patients who were hyperglycaemic on large doses of subcutaneously injected insulin (120–3000 units). Glycaemic control was improved by up to 48 hours intravenous insulin infusion using lower doses (50–63 units). Freidenberg et al[35] extended the intravenous infusion period to 1–6 months in 4 female type 1 diabetic patients with subcutaneous insulin resistance and recurrent DKA. A portable pump was used with delivery via a subcutaneously tunnelled silastic cannula into the superior vena cava. Infusion was considered necessary for survival in these patients, but was associated with significant complications, including phlebitis, thrombosis, septicaemia and catheter breakage.

A similar disappointing experience was noted by our own group when treating 5 CSII-unresponsive brittle diabetic subjects by CIVII via an indwelling central venous catheter.[36] Over treatment periods of between 3 and 16 months, the lives of these patients continued to be disrupted by frequent hospital admissions and, except for short periods, there was continued hyperglycaemia, erratic swings in blood glucose concentration and ketosis. In several cases (although not all), interference with treatment was detected, including disconnection of catheters at the pump, removal of catheters from the vein despite stitching to the skin under occlusive dressings and suspected dilution of the pump insulin with tap water (subsequently admitted by the patient). All of the patients had complications of intravenous infusion such as septicaemia, intermittent catheter blockage and dislodged catheters.

A case has also been described of a 23-year-old type 1 diabetic woman who was massively resistant to insulin administered by all routes and infusion regimens, including CIVII.[37] Up to 20 000 units per day of insulin were required by CIVII (via a Hickman catheter tunnelled into the subclavian vein and then into the right atrium), which was maintained for 4 years. Inappropriately low plasma free insulin concentrations during high-dose CIVII (<60 mU/l) suggested rapid clearance of insulin from the circulation.

Intermittent intravenous insulin infusion

The studies of CIVII described above have used continuous insulin infusion. An alternative intravenous strategy administers insulin as a series of pulses, with the intent of inducing greater hepatic activation. Aoki et al[38] reported on 20 type 1 diabetic subjects with wide swings in blood glucose concentration and/or frequent hypoglycaemia who were treated by intermittent intravenous insulin for between 7 and 71 months. The regimen consisted of 7–10 2–unit insulin pulses given over 60 minutes, three times daily into a peripheral vein, with maintenance therapy on one day per week. The mean number of severe hypoglycaemic episodes was reduced from 3.0 to 0.1 episodes per month and the HbA_{1c} from 8.5 to 7.0%. Unfortunately, the study had no randomly allocated control group treated by optimized injection therapy and there was no comparison with an established continuous infusion regimen such as CSII, so interpretation is difficult. Nevertheless, this approach deserves further study.

Continuous intraperitoneal insulin infusion

Continuous intraperitoneal insulin infusion (CIPII) from an external pump has achieved temporary improvement in control and reduced insulin dosages in some CSII-unresponsive patients with recurrent ketoacidosis,[39,40] but control tends to deteriorate subsequently and peritonitis is a complication. For example, Husband et al[40] treated 6 such patients by CIPII for between 3 and 12 months (mean 7 months); complications included catheter dislodgement, abscesses at the catheter tip and catheter blockage. Whereas there was short-term near normoglycaemia (mean blood glucose 5.8 mmol/l), the mean HbA_{1c} was 13.3% at 3 months and 12.2% at 6 months CIPII. Some patients spent less time in hospital during CIPII, indicating a partial success for the treatment. Gill et al[25] have stated that CIPII can be spectacularly successful in the occasional patient and we have recently managed a type 1 diabetic subject on CIPII who was previously well controlled for many years on CSII and then developed continuous ketosis, which could not be abolished with CSII without inducing hypoglycaemia. CIPII has produced acceptable control without ketosis in this patient for more than a year.

279

Continuous intramuscular insulin infusion

The intramuscular route has had some short-term success in improving control in CSII-unresponsive subjects but has not proved a practicable long-term option. We found that 5 out of 6 brittle type 1 diabetic patients with recurrent DKA were improved by continuous intramuscular insulin infusion (CIMII) into the deltoid muscle for up to 9 days (mean blood glucose 13.6 ± 5.8 mmol/l during CSII and 7.7 ± 2.6 mmol/l during CIMII). Outpatient studies have been performed in relatively few patients and have been complicated by the difficulty of securing the cannula and fibrosis at the insertion point.

Implantable insulin infusion pumps

A limited number of type 1 diabetic patients with extreme resistance to subcutaneous insulin but relatively normal sensitivity to intravenous insulin have been improved by implantable insulin pump therapy with either intravenous or intraperitoneal insulin delivery.[41–45]

A number of case reports on implantable pump therapy of brittle diabetes performed in the 1980s indicated impressive responses in some, with rapid institution of near normoglycaemia and reduction in hospital admissions.[41–43] A more modern audit in a larger group of 33 patients in The Netherlands treated by the Medtronic MiniMed implanted intraperitoneal pump was somewhat less impressive.[45] Although hospital admissions were reduced in a subgroup of 20 patients in whom this was a clinical problem, the mean HbA_{1c} on pump therapy was 9.0%, there was a relatively low quality of life and a number of patients had psychiatric symptoms, although this probably reflected pre-existing psychosocial disorder. Unfortunately, there was no pre-pump assessment of quality of life or psychiatric status in these patients. Also, the authors did not report technical failures and complications of implantable insulin pump therapy, which in non-brittle patients include insulin underdelivery caused by aggregation of insulin in the pump or catheter blockage caused by fibrin clots or omental encapsulation.[46,47] These problems have significantly impaired routine clinical use of implantable pumps in non-brittle diabetic subjects.

Although it is possible that this treatment bypasses an abnormality of subcutaneous insulin handling, it is equally the case that the inaccessibility of the implanted pump simply offers less opportunity for tampering and interference of diabetes management by the patient, considered by many to be the most usual cause of the recurrent DKA-insulin resistance type of brittle diabetes.[28,48]

The dawn phenomenon

The dawn phenomenon is a marked rise in blood glucose concentration in the few hours preceding breakfast; it is thought to be caused by a combination of waning of the preceding night's long-acting insulin injection and an increase in insulin resistance due to growth hormone surges during the night.[49,50] CSII is a recognized management strategy for the dawn phenomenon, as the basal rate can be preset automatically to increase during the night and counter the fasting hyperglycaemia. In practice, the dawn phenomenon is an unusual indication for CSII and, amongst patients treated by CSII with a single basal rate, a significant pre-breakfast blood glucose rise is rare.[51]

New long-acting insulins with a flatter insulin profile during the night, such as insulin glargine, may be helpful in managing the dawn phenomenon without resort to pump therapy but little is known about how insulin glargine compares with CSII. Preliminary studies indicate that CSII is still more effective at controlling fasting hyperglycaemia than insulin glargine,[52] although individual patients may respond to the analogue more favourably.

Diabetic pregnancy and pre-pregnancy

Hypoglycaemia can be more frequent during pregnancy than at any other time of the diabetic woman's life. There are several factors that contribute to this,[53] including general attempts to improve control by lowering the average glycaemic level, passive diffusion of glucose across the placenta to the fetus, lowered availability of the gluconeogenic amino acid alanine and reduced counter-regulatory hormone release in response to induced hypoglycaemia. The tendency to

281

hypoglycaemia can also be aggravated by decreased food intake secondary to morning sickness.

There is no evidence from randomized controlled trials that CSII achieves a lower mean blood glucose concentration than multiple insulin injections in unselected type 1 diabetic subjects during pregnancy.[54–56] However, as with non-pregnant subjects, individuals who are not well controlled on optimized injection regimens because of frequent hypoglycaemia can be improved. A non-randomized study has shown about a 70% reduction in severe hypoglycaemia in pregnant women with type 1 diabetes treated by CSII, compared with multiple insulin injections.[57] Ideally, strict blood glucose control should be achieved before conception and diabetic women wishing to become pregnant should be considered for CSII if optimized injection therapy fails to maintain satisfactory metabolic control.

Poor control in type 2 diabetes receiving oral hypoglycaemic agents or insulin injections

More than a decade ago, Jennings et al[58] reported a group of type 2 diabetic patients who were poorly controlled while receiving sulphonylureas and then randomly allocated to either twice-daily short-acting and isophane insulin or to CSII. Fasting and mean blood glucose concentrations and HbA_{1c} percentage were all significantly lower in the group treated by CSII. Although this study did not compare CSII with modern optimized injection therapy in type 2 diabetes, it hinted at a possible use for pumps in this type of diabetes. Surprisingly, it is only in the last couple of years that researchers have returned to evaluating the role of CSII in type 2 diabetes. The conclusions are uncertain and the effectiveness of CSII in tablet-failed patients seems not to have been explored further.

In one study, severely obese type 2 patients with resistance to insulin by injection (>1 unit/kg/day) who were transferred to CSII for 40 weeks enjoyed a mean HbA_{1c} fall from 12.3 to 9.6%.[59] In another report by the same group,[60] HbA_{1c} was comparable after random allocation to CSII or multiple injections in previously poorly controlled obese type 2 patients. This suggests that CSII and multiple injections are both superior to conventional injection regimens in the treatment of type 2 diabetes.

Pancreas and islet cell transplantation

Islet transplantation, although less invasive and costly than pancreas transplantation, has had, until recently, a poor record of achieving insulin independence in type 1 diabetes. However, the so-called Edmonton protocol, first reported in the year 2000,[2] has allowed a remarkable success rate for islet transplantation in recent years, with 100% of the original patients and 85% of a subsequent follow-up[61] achieving insulin independence. The main features of the new protocol are transplantation of an adequate islet cell mass, a potent steroid-free immunosuppressive regimen, immediate transplantation of freshly isolated islets and careful selection of patients without renal failure.

The indications for islet transplantation used by the Edmonton group included brittle diabetes and hypoglycaemia unawareness despite optimization of insulin therapy, although no definitions of brittle diabetes were given.[62] Diabetic instability was resolved in all of the patients, with only 3 of the 12 having post-transplant diabetes. Suitable candidates for islet-alone transplantation are given as those with two episodes of severe hypoglycaemia in the previous 6 months, and self-monitored blood glucose values during optimized insulin therapy of <2.5–3.0 mmol/l, without symptoms. In the most recent report of 32 consecutive patients treated in Edmonton, all patients had complete correction of hypoglycaemia (85% insulin-free at 1 year).[61]

The potential risks of islet implantation through the percutaneous intraportal route include bleeding from the liver surface, portal vein thrombosis and the longer-term risks of immunosuppression (drug-specific side effects such as nephrotoxicity, life-threatening infection and post-transplant malignancy). The complications and risks of the Edmonton protocol in follow-up to date are reasonably small, although of course the long-term effects are unknown. With more experience of this new therapy, we may soon reach the position where, in highly selected individuals with severe brittle diabetes unresponsive to other management strategies, the benefits of islet cell transplantation may exceed any risks.

Although the criteria for pancreas transplantation alone at some centres include 'hyperlabile' diabetes with episodes of ketoacidosis, severe and frequent hypoglycaemia and impaired quality of life,[63] the procedure has not been rigorously tested as a treatment for brittle diabetes; however, occasional positive case reports have been recorded.[64,65] It is likely to be superseded by islet transplantation.

Conclusions

CSII has emerged as an effective management strategy for at least one major class of type 1 diabetic patient with difficult control: those with frequent unpredictable hypoglycaemia in spite of best attempts to improve control with modern optimized insulin injection regimens. Although frequent hypoglycaemia is also an indication for islet cell transplantation and first results with the Edmonton protocol show that this problem resolves after transplantation, it is likely that CSII should be the first alternative treatment tested.

In those with recurrent ketoacidosis/insulin resistance, overall glycaemic control does not usually improve with CSII, although recent studies indicate that the number of admissions to hospital can be significantly reduced in some patients. Simple CSII regimens based on basal rates without prandial boosts may be worth testing.

When there is life-threatening brittle diabetes with recurrent DKA, unresponsive to CSII, continuous intraperitoneal infusion should be considered. Totally implanted insulin pumps have achieved some success with such patients, particularly in dramatically reducing hospital stays, but the glycaemic control may be only slightly improved (to an HbA$_{1c}$ of about 9%). Nevertheless, implanted pumps are costly, invasive and have significant complications, which at the moment restricts their wider use. Islet cell transplantation clearly has potential in this class of brittle diabetes, but has yet to be evaluated.

References

1. Pickup J, Keen H. Continuous subcutaneous insulin infusion at 25 years. Evidence base for the expanding use of insulin pump therapy in type 1 diabetes. Diabetes Care 2002; 25: 593–8.
2. Shapiro AMJ, Lakey JRT, Ryan EA et al. Islet transplantation in seven patients with Type 1 diabetes mellitus using a glucocorticoid-free immunosuppressive regimen. N Engl J Med 2000; 343: 230–8.
3. Pickup JC. Alternative forms of insulin delivery. In: Pickup JC, Williams G, eds, Textbook of diabetes, 3rd edn. Blackwell Publishers, Oxford, 2003, pp 44.1–44.15.
4. Kauffman FR, Halvorson M, Miller D et al. Insulin pump therapy in type 1 pediatric patients: now and into the year 2000. Diab Metab Res Rev 1999; 15: 338–52.
5. Locke DR, Rigg LA. Hypoglycemic coma associated with subcutaneous insulin infusion by portable pump. Diabetes Care 1981; 4: 389–91.
6. Giacomet AC. Hypoglycemic coma associated with CSII. Diabetes Care 1983; 6: 316–17.
7. Dahl-Jørgensen K, Brinchman-Hansen O, Hanssen KF et al. Effect of near-normoglycaemia for two years on the progression of early diabetic retinopathy: the Oslo Study. Br Med J 1986; 293: 1195–9.
8. Bending JJ, Pickup JC, Keen H. Frequency of diabetic ketoacidosis and hypoglycemic coma during treatment with continuous subcutaneous insulin infusion. Am J Med 1985; 79: 685–91.
9. Bode BW, Steed RD, Davidson PC. Reduction in severe hypoglycemia with long-term continuous subcutaneous insulin infusion in type 1 diabetes. Diabetes Care 1996; 19: 324–7.
10. Boland EA, Grey M, Oesterle A, Fredrickson L, Tamborlane WV. Continuous subcutaneous insulin infusion. A new way to lower risk of severe hypoglycemia, improve metabolic control, and enhance coping in adolescents with type 1 diabetes. Diabetes Care 1999; 22: 1779–84.
11. Haardt MJ, Berne C, Dorange C, Slama G, Selam J-L. Efficacy and indications of CSII revisited: the Hôtel Dieu cohort. Diabet Med 1997; 14: 407–8.
12. Pickup J, Mattock M, Kerry S. Glycaemic control with continuous subcutaneous insulin infusion compared to intensive insulin injection therapy in type 1 diabetes: meta-analysis of randomised controlled trials. Br Med J 2002; 324: 705–8.
13. Lauritzen T, Pramming S, Deckert T, Binder C. Pharmacokinetics of continuous subcutaneous insulin infusion. Diabetologia 1983; 24: 326–9.
14. Cryer PE. Iatrogenic hypoglycemia as a cause of hypoglycemia associated autonomic failure in IDDM: a vicious circle. Diabetes 1992; 41: 255–60.
15. Heller SR. Hypoglycaemia and diabetes. In: Pickup JC, Williams G, eds,

Textbook of diabetes, 3rd edn. Blackwell Publishers, Oxford, 2003, pp 33.1–33.19.

16. Fanelli CG, Epifano L, Rambotti et al. Meticulous prevention of hypoglycemia normalizes the glycemic thresholds and magnitude of most neuroendocrine responses to, symptoms of, and cognitive function during hypoglycemia in intensively treated patients with short-term IDDM. Diabetes 1993; 42: 1683–9.

17. Cranston I, Lomas J, Maran A, Macdonald I, Amiel SA. Restoration of hypoglycaemia awareness in patients with long-duration insulin-dependent diabetes. Lancet 1994; 344: 283–7.

18. Dagogo-Jack S, Rattarasarn C, Cryer PE. Reversal of hypoglycemia unawareness, but not defective glucose counterregulation, in IDDM. Diabetes 1994; 43: 1426–34.

19. Kanc K, Janssen MM, Keulen ETP et al. Substitution of night-time continuous subcutaneous insulin infusion therapy for bedtime NPH insulin in a multiple injection regimen improves counterregulatory hormonal responses and warning symptoms of hypoglycaemia in IDDM. Diabetologia 1998; 41: 322–9.

20. Hirsch IB, Farkas-Hirsch R, Cryer PE. Continuous subcutaneous insulin infusion for the treatment of diabetic patients with hypoglycemia unawareness. Diab Nutr Metab 1991; 4: 41–3.

21. Prendergast JJ, Aubrey W. Severe autonomic neuropathy treated with subcutaneous insulin infusion. Diabetes Care 1996; 19: 90.

22. Lauritzen T, Frost-Larsen K, Larsen HW, Deckert T. The Steno Study Group: two-year experience with continuous subcutaneous insulin infusion in relation to retinopathy and neuropathy. Diabetes 1985; 34(suppl 3): 74–9.

23. Horowitz M, Fraser R. Disordered gastric motor function in diabetes mellitus. Diabetologia 1994; 37: 543–51.

24. Pickup JC, Williams G, Johns P, Keen H. Clinical features of brittle diabetic patients unresponsive to optimised subcutaneous insulin therapy. Diabetes Care 1983; 6: 279–84.

25. Gill GV, Walford S, Alberti KGMM. Brittle diabetes – present concepts. Diabetologia 1985; 28: 579–89.

26. Gill GV, Lucas S, Kent LA. Prevalence and characteristics of brittle diabetes in Britain. Quart J Med 1996; 89: 839–43.

27. Pickup JC, Home PD, Bilous RW, Keen H, Alberti KGMM. Management of severely brittle diabetes by continuous subcutaneous and intramuscular insulin infusions: evidence for a defect in subcutaneous insulin absorption. Br Med J 1981; 282: 347–50.

28. Schade DS, Drumm DA, Duckworth WC, Eaton RP. The etiology of incapacitating brittle diabetes. Diabetes Care 1985; 8: 12–20.

29. Nathan DM. Successful treatment of extremely brittle, insulin-dependent diabetes with a novel subcutaneous insulin pump regimen. Diabetes Care 1982; 5: 105–10.

30. Steindel BS, Roe TR, Costin G et al. Continuous subcutaneous insulin infusion (CSII) in children and adolescents with poorly controlled type 1 diabetes mellitus. Diab Res Clin Pract 1995; 27: 199–204.

31. Blackett PR. Insulin pump treatment for recurrent ketoacidosis in adolescence. Diabetes Care 1995; 18: 881–2.

32. Chantelau E, Spraul M, Mühlhauser I, Gause R, Berger M. Long-term safety, efficacy and side effects of continuous subcutaneous insulin infusion treatment for type 1 (insulin-dependent) diabetes mellitus: a one centre experience. Diabetologia 1989; 32: 421–6.

33. Kamoi K. Good long-term quality of life without diabetic complications with 20 years continuous subcutaneous insulin infusion therapy in a brittle diabetic elderly patient. Diabetes Care 2002; 25: 402–4.

34. Dandona P, Healey F, Foster M et al. Low-dose insulin infusions in diabetic patients with high insulin requirements. Lancet 1978; ii: 283–5.

35. Freidenberg GR, White N, Cataland S et al. Diabetes responsive to intravenous but not subcutaneous insulin: effectiveness of aprotinin. N Engl J Med 1981; 305: 363–8.

36. Williams G, Pickup JC, Keen H. Continuous intravenous insulin infusion in the management of brittle diabetes: etiologic and therapeutic implications. Diabetes Care 1985: 8: 21–7.

37. Williams G, Pickup JC, Keen H. Massive insulin resistance apparently due to rapid clearance of circulating insulin. Am J Med 1987; 82: 1247–52.

38. Aoki TT, Benbarka MM, Okimura MC et al. Long-term intermittent intravenous insulin therapy and type 1 diabetes mellitus. Lancet 1993; 342: 515–18.

39. Pozza G, Spotti D, Micossi P et al. Long-term continuous intraperitoneal insulin treatment in brittle diabetes. Br Med J 1983; 286: 255–6.

40. Husband DJ, Marshall SM, Walford S et al. Continuous intraperitoneal insulin infusion in the management of severely brittle diabetes – a metabolic and clinical comparison with intravenous insulin. Diab Med 1984; 1: 99–104.

41. Campbell IW, Kritz H, Najemnik C et al. Treatment of type 1 diabetic with subcutaneous insulin resistance by a totally implantable insulin infusion device ("Infusaid"). Diab Res 1984; 1: 83–8.

42. Buchwald H, Chute EP, Goldenberg FJ et al. Implantable infusion pump management of insulin resistant diabetes mellitus. Ann Surg 1985; 202: 278–82.

43. Gill GV, Husband DJ, Wright PD et al. The management of severe brittle diabetes with "Infusaid" implantable pumps. Diab Res 1986; 3: 135–7.

44. Wood DF, Goodchild K, Guillou P, Thomas DJ, Johnston DG. Management of 'brittle diabetes' with a preprogrammable implanted insulin pump delivering intraperitoneal insulin. Br Med J 1990; 301: 1143–4.

45. DeVries JH, Eskes SA, Snoek FJ et al. Continuous intraperitoneal insulin

infusion in patients with "brittle" diabetes: favourable effects on glycaemic control and hospital stay. Diab Med 2002; 19: 496–501.

46. Renard E, Baldet P, Picot M-C et al. Catheter complications associated with implantable systems for peritoneal insulin delivery. Diabetes Care 1995; 18: 300–6.

47. Renard E, Bouteleau S, Jacques-Apostol D et al. Insulin underdelivery from implanted pumps using peritoneal route. Diabetes Care 1996; 19: 812–17.

48. Tattersall RB. Brittle diabetes revisited. The Third Arnold Bloom Lecture. Diab Med 1997; 14: 99–110.

49. Campbell PJ, Bolli G, Cryer PE, Gerich JE. Pathogenesis of the dawn phenomenon in patients with insulin-dependent diabetes mellitus. N Engl J Med 1985; 312: 1473–9.

50. Perriello G, De Feo P, Fanelli C, Santeusanio F, Bolli G. Nocturnal spikes of growth hormone secretion cause the dawn phenomenon in type 1 (insulin-dependent) diabetes mellitus by decreasing hepatic (and extra-hepatic) sensitivity to insulin in the absence of insulin waning. Diabetologia 1990; 33: 52–9.

51. Bending JJ, Pickup JC, Collins ACG, Keen H. Rarity of a marked dawn phenomenon in diabetic subjects treated by continuous subcutaneous insulin infusion. Diabetes Care 1985; 8: 28–33.

52. Armstrong DU, King AB. Basal insulin: continuous glucose monitoring reveals less over-night hypoglycemia with continuous subcutaneous insulin infusion than with glargine. Diabetes 2002; 51(suppl 2): 92A.

53. Jornsay DL. Continuous subcutaneous insulin infusion (CSII) therapy during pregnancy. Diabetes Spectrum 1998; 11: 26–32.

54. Coustan DR, Reece E, Sherwin RS et al. A randomised clinical trial of the insulin pump vs. intensive conventional therapy in diabetic pregnancies. JAMA 1986; 255: 631–6.

55. Carta Q, Meriggi E, Trossarelli GF et al. Continuous subcutaneous insulin infusion versus intensive conventional insulin therapy in type I and type II diabetic pregnancy. Diabete Metabolisme (Paris) 1986; 12: 121–9.

56. Nosari I, Maglio ML, Lepore G, Pagani G. Is continuous subcutaneous insulin infusion more effective than intensive conventional insulin therapy in the treatment of pregnant diabetic women? Diab Nutr Metab 1993; 6: 33–7.

57. Frias JP, Gottlieb PA, Mackenzie T et al. Better glycemic control and less severe hypoglycemia in pregnant women with type 1 diabetes treated with continuous subcutaneous insulin infusion. Diabetes 2002; 51(suppl 2): 431A.

58. Jennings AM, Lewis KS, Murdoch S et al. Randomized trial comparing continuous subcutaneous insulin infusion and conventional insulin therapy in type II diabetic patients poorly controlled with sulfonylureas. Diabetes Care 1991; 14: 738–44.

59. Wainstein J, Metzger M, Wexler ID et al. The use of continuous insulin delivery systems in severely insulin-resistant patients. Diabetes Care 2001; 24: 1299.

60. Wainstein J, Metzger M, Menuchin O et al. Insulin pump therapy versus multiple daily injections in obese type 2 patients. Diabetologia 2001; 44(suppl 1): 26A.

61. Shapiro AMJ, Ryan EA, Paty BW, Lakey JRT. Pancreas and islet transplantation. In: Pickup JC, Williams G, eds, Textbook of diabetes, 3rd edn. Blackwell Publishers, Oxford, 2003, pp 72.1–72.18.

62. Ryan EA, Lakey JRT, Rajotte RV et al. Clinical outcomes and insulin secretion after islet transplantation with the Edmonton protocol. Diabetes 2001; 50: 710–19.

63. Hakim NS. Recent developments and future prospects in pancreatic and islet transplantation. Diabetes Obesity Metab 2001; 3: 9–15.

64. DuToit DF, Heydenrych JJ, Coetzee AR, Weight M. Pancreatic transplantation in a patient with severe insulin resistance. South Afr Med J 1988; 73: 723–5.

65. Robinson ACJ, Pacy P, Kearney T et al. Pancreatic transplantation in "brittle" diabetes mellitus – a case report. Diabet Med 1996; 13(suppl 7): S11.

chapter 14

Living with brittle diabetes

A patient

Living with brittle diabetes is hassle and hell. When I was first diagnosed it all seemed very strange. I was in hospital for about a fortnight and then I was out in the big wide world trying to come to terms with what was happening to my body. I felt a failure. A failure to my parents, my brother and my sister. In some way I felt I had let them down with something I had no control over – my pancreas not producing enough insulin for me to lead a 'normal' life. I was angry. Also, I felt afraid. Afraid especially of hypos. Having visions of ending up in hospital through going into a coma by taking too much insulin and not waking up in the morning. To this day I still haven't come to terms with the fact that I may go hypo in the middle of the night, and my husband may not be able to wake me up to give me sugar of some description – after 23 years of having the wretched disease.

In the first few years of being diabetic, I rebelled against myself by eating all the wrong sorts of food and not taking insulin, in the hope that one day it would all go away. The honeymoon may well be over for myself, but it is still at the back of my mind when I am giving my evening dose of insulin.

I was diagnosed when I was 14 years of age. I had many hospital admissions with ketoacidosis because I couldn't get used to the idea that I had to punish (or so it seemed) myself with twice-daily injections. I had done nothing wrong to have been diagnosed with diabetes. One nurse took great delight in telling me that I would have to have injections for the rest of my life. Well that is what she thought! In those days, I manipulated myself into going into ketoacidosis through not taking enough insulin. I was admitted on numerous occasions, and at 16 years of age I was transferred from the paediatric clinic to an adult clinic nearer to my home. Within 2 months I was back in hospital through poor control. This scared me a little, as I was now the 'baby' on the ward. A lot of the staff used to say, 'poor you – you have not had much of a life apart from being in and out of hospital'. After a 3-month stay in the local hospital, the doctors thought it best that I went to a specialized centre for diabetes. I was sent to a London hospital at the age of 17 years.

This was really like stepping into the big league. I was far away from home and family. My dad used to visit on a Sunday with my brother and sister, and mum came to see me on a Wednesday. People used to think my mum and dad were divorced because they travelled on different days! How wrong could they be, as actually it all brought my family even closer. Down in London I was petrified that the doctors would see that I had my finger on the self-destruct button. I had a central venous (CVP) line inserted, but I managed to get water into the insulin syringe connected to the line. Result – blood sugars through the roof, and occasional septicaemia! I saw a psychiatrist whilst in London to try and see why I was always wanting to manipulate my blood sugars and send myself into ketoacidosis, but I couldn't open up to him. I was now getting very clever into tricking the doctors about watering down the insulin. And yet, I *was* really becoming insulin resistant – hand on heart (to this day I am still on over 135 units of insulin each day).

After spending close on 18 months in London I came home on intravenous insulin via a CVP line, and an insulin pump around my waist. Again, the temptation came, and I ended up being admitted to a local hospital with septicaemia (my fault again, but I did used to get frightened at home in case my family couldn't cope with me). I again felt a failure to them, yet I was tearing the family apart. Amazingly, they never doubted me, and always believed me when I said that I had nothing to do with causing the admissions. After spending many months in the local hospital, the doctors again sent me away from home. Newcastle was my destination this time. Here I spent 2 years in hospital with various insulins tried upon me and CVP lines again used (to date I have had 20 CVP lines and 12 peritoneal lines used). The doctors in Newcastle were more determined to get me sorted out. I had fat biopsies, blood sugars tested every hour for a day or two, and at one stage I was even linked up to a machine called an 'artificial pancreas'!

Though in the early days of being diagnosed it brought myself and my family together closer, being so far away in these specialist centres put a strain on the family. I met other brittle diabetic patients from around the country and sometimes 'swapped' ideas of how to cheat the system – trying to defy what the doctors were doing in attempting to bring our diabetes under control. Every sort of external insulin pump had been tried on me with no success. Being so unstable – in my mind as well as my body – I was eventually operated on to implant an insulin pump ("Infusaid") into my abdominal wall. With this, I wasn't able to dilute the insulin with water and I learnt the hard way of coping with diabetes. It had its advantages though – no more needles (except the one to fill the Infusaid every 3 weeks). This was a great relief for me as I hated injections and I still do. The cannula from the pump was led into my peritoneum, and it felt strange that I was able to lead a normal way of life. Diabetes was no longer a major factor. I could eat practically what I wanted. However, after 2 years had passed the Infusaid began to malfunction, so I was yet again admitted to hospital where an operation to take out the pump was performed. Back to the dreaded injections was now the only way forward.

With brittle diabetes, although insulin is injected it is not always absorbed, and huge doses of insulin may be required. But manipulation is also the name of the game! People with diabetes who do cheat the system either draw air into their syringes or bottles, or put water into the insulin. Quite often septicaemia is inevitable, because the water put into the syringe is not sterile! After many CVP lines, I have both my subclavian veins blocked. This was why peritoneal lines were then used, but this time water in the pump caused peritonitis. Doctors often don't believe a patient when they say that they have had their insulin, if their blood glucose level is high; and may accuse the patient of cheating on their diet or not injecting insulin. They are often quite right! A lot of the patients I have met – especially in London and Newcastle – cheated the system because they could not accept the fact that they had a disease that was not going to go away, and that they felt a failure to themselves and family. The question 'Why me?' is always asked, and there is never a reason or answer to it.

I have had almost every combination of insulin treatments known, but when I think of all the treatments, four daily injections is the best for me. I am older and wiser to the complications of diabetes now, as I have experienced one or two of them – in particular retinopathy and neuropathy. The treatment of retinopathy is not very pleasant. Anaesthetic drops are put into the eye, along with drops to enlarge the pupil, so that the doctor can see the retina more clearly and laser the blood vessels that are leaking or bleeding. My eyes are always sore after laser treatment. I have notified the DVLA of my retinopathy and up to now I have had no problems renewing my driving licence (I usually get a licence for 3 years). Also, I only now attend my diabetic clinic on a yearly basis but can, if need be, contact the diabetic nurses if I am having any problems. I am fortunate that I have a very caring husband, and after we had our little boy I gave up work (or put another way I was signed off due to ill health). I don't miss it and am pleased that I am at home looking after my children the best way I can. I have two beautiful children, but the pregnancies were far from straightforward.

With me being a brittle diabetic, the doctors were very cautious in looking after me. I got to 12 weeks in my first pregnancy when I saw the consultant, and admission to the antenatal ward loomed. My diabetes was extremely unstable needing lots more insulin, and some days I had to have insulin every 2 hours. I also had to have lots of laser treatment to my eyes as my retinopathy progressed in the wrong direction. I had scans every 2 weeks, and at 31 weeks I was given steroid injections to try and help my baby's lungs develop. My little boy was born at 32 weeks by Caesarean section and weighed 5 lb 12 oz. He was quite poorly in the special baby care unit – needing to be placed on a ventilator for the first 10 days of his life. These were frightening times for my husband and myself, yet it didn't put me off having another child. The consultant tried to talk me out of this, but I was determined that my little boy was not going to be an only child. Some people said I was stupid in trying for another, but I always wanted two children. When my first child was 2 years old, I fell pregnant again. This time I only got to 8 weeks gestation and admission was necessary. I stayed yet again in hospital for the rest of my pregnancy. At 4 months I had another CVP line inserted and again I developed septicaemia – not through any fault of my own (I wouldn't dream of hurting my baby in any shape or form). The diabetologist and obstetrician discussed the option of abortion, but no way! I went on to deliver, again very early (33 weeks gestation), a beautiful baby girl who weighed 5 lb 6 oz. Again, she needed special baby care assistance, but was not in as much danger as our little boy. Both of my children have come to no harm, even though I had difficult pregnancies. At the delivery of my little girl, my obstetrician tied my fallopian tubes (with my permission). He said that if I was going to have any more children, he would resign!

Brittle diabetes can have psychological complications. I suffer from depression and I would say that diabetes and depression go 'hand-in-hand'. After the birth of my little girl I suffered from terrible post-natal depression, which meant I had a very long stay in a psychiatric ward. I do not remember the first 9 months of my little girl's life, as during this time I needed to have electroconvulsive therapy (ECT). I am still on antidepressants and tranquillizers. If I become very depressed, my diabetes is not a priority and gets neglected because I cannot be bothered with life in general. In the past I have refused insulin when depressed, and have even been forced to have it under a Mental Health Act section. As mentioned before, I saw a psychiatrist in London and also in Newcastle. In Newcastle I attended a young people's unit for psychiatric problems 3 times a week. I hated it. We used to play games to try and sort out our own problems, and we had group therapy to say how we felt. I would never 'open up' to anyone that was to do with this unit for young people. I know that on discharge from Newcastle, the psychiatrist saw my parents and suggested that I had a spell in a local psychiatric ward, as I was 'institutionalized' with having the best part of my adolescent years in hospital. My parents objected to this suggestion however, and I returned home.

With having the insulin pump implanted, manipulating my diabetes was out of the question. However, I was admitted to our local hospital with appendicitis, and when the diabetes consultant saw me, he knew that there was something troubling me. I used to lie on my bed and stare into space, not taking any notice of anyone else. I refused to talk, sleep, eat or drink; so my consultant referred me to a local psychiatrist. He thought I was clinically depressed (he was right). Thankfully, I seem to be on the right type of medication now, and I also have a CPN (community psychiatric nurse) who visits me every fortnight to make sure things are OK (which they seem to be at the moment).

I would like to say that I am a bit more responsible nowadays and try to look after myself. My marriage and children have had a lot to do with this. As a family we go away at weekends to our caravan in Wales. This time together is very precious, as my husband works away a lot, so we make good use of our weekends together.

I still remember the bad times of the past, however. During the dark days of my long admission in Newcastle, I found a poem somewhere, and changed it by putting the word 'diabetes' in at certain places. It still sums up what I feel about having diabetes.

I have done what most men do,
and pushed it out of my mind.
But I can't forget if I wanted to,
diabetes trotting behind.

Day after day, the whole day through,
wherever my road inclined,
diabetes said 'I am coming with you',
and trotted along behind.

Now I must go by some other round
which I shall never find.
Somewhere that does not carry the sound
of diabetes trotting behind.

Index

Note: references to figures are indicated by 'f' and references to tables by 't' when they fall on pages not covered by the text reference

UNIVERSITY OF WOLVERHAMPTON
LEARNING & INFORMATION SERVICES